Crisis Pregnancy Centers:

The Birth Of A Grassroots Movement

Terry Ianora

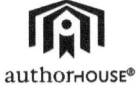

authorHOUSE®

AuthorHouse™
1663 Liberty Drive
Bloomington, IN 47403
www.authorhouse.com
Phone: 1-800-839-8640

First published by AuthorHouse 6/9/2009

ISBN: 978-1-4389-8572-5 (e)
ISBN: 978-1-4389-8570-1 (sc)
ISBN: 978-1-4389-8571-8 (hc)

Printed in the United States of America
Bloomington, Indiana

This book is printed on acid-free paper.

Dedication

To the Moms who, against so many ferocious pressures to abort their unplanned pregnancies, carried their precious babies to term. They are the heroes.

Table of Contents

Acknowledgement

Thanks to Kathy O'Boyle, my shift partner at the 1st Way office, who encouraged me to write this story. Hers was the difficult task of deciphering my handwritten draft over the course of an entire year. In the moments when I wanted to give up the work she was always there presenting me with yet another skillfully typed chapter, a verification that the work was actually taking shape.

Thanks to Molly Peterson, the editor, with her intuitive skill at discerning what I truly wanted to say. She was another gift from God. I cannot resist the analogy of juxtaposing this developing of this history with the gestation of a baby. For, in reality, Molly became pregnant at the start of this work and it left her computer upon the birth of her baby, Felix.

I also send my heartfelt thanks to my fearless leader, Denise Cocciolone, President of the National Life Center, who has labored for almost 40 years along with the founder, Louise Summerhill, to spare women the trauma of abortion by bringing the idea of "alternatives to abortion" to its proper place on this earth.

Thanks to the women directors of their centers who had the courage and vision to contribute their memories to this story of the pro-life pregnancy service movement.

Preface

Love. That used to be a word to describe the very basic human emotion that led to self-giving and sacrifice. How far away from the life-giving and happiness producing reality was the relationship experienced by Wendy. Brushing aside a stray bit of hair from her forehead, Wendy sat alone in the 1st Way office one sunny afternoon. She had been riding her bike, she said, when she noticed the 1st Way sign. Free pregnancy tests, free ultrasound, so she decided that it was time to get some answers to her many physical symptoms. Her story is a sad one: on her own at age 15, Wendy drifted into a romantic relationship wish a school friend. When she found out she was pregnant there seemed to be little help to carry a baby. Her parents, she said, had their own problems. Out of this necessity, Wendy turned to abortion. In her own words, it was a terrible experience. From then on she drifted, making some money as a cook, living with different friends.

At 23 she was involved with a man whose own family had been blighted by abortion. Living at her boyfriends parents home she had heard many times how much he resented the fact that he had no siblings. It was due, he said, to the multiple abortions of his mother. But, despite this attitude, he let her know that he did not feel ready to be a father if she should turn up pregnant. All this Wendy related to the volunteer in a matter-of-fact manner. But this volunteer could sense that this was a young woman, who although deeply hurt by youthful hardships, possessed an inner strength.

When the test came back positive, Wendy began to finger a small hole in the sleeve of her sweater. She looked up and let out a sigh. Was she reliving her past abortion experience? Something kept

Wendy transfixed to the spot in front of the lab table. The volunteer took Wendy's hand. Together they moved and sat down on a couch. Gently, carefully, the volunteer spoke to Wendy about the many opportunities and aids that were available to pregnant women in Eugene. Even if she could not stay in her boyfriend's home there were homes to take their place. Her medical and prenatal bills would be covered and she could have the faithful friendship of women such as herself all through the pregnancy and beyond. Wendy gazed at the table at her elbow, where actual life-sized models of babies in various states of development were displayed. Then, she asked if she could use the telephone. It was her boyfriend's number. Yes, he agreed to come to the office where, together, they could talk matters over with the volunteer. An appointment was made for both to view their baby on the ultrasound. A shy smile replaced the tense look in Wendy's eyes. This could turn out for the better.

Introduction

In the early morning a woman is boarding a plane, destination Minneapolis, Minnesota. She is anxious and hopeful. The person she is to meet may have the answer to her burning desire to perform some personal service to save the unborn from the scourge of abortion. The meeting between Louise Summerhill and Denise Cocciolone turns out to be an historic one--an alliance between two women. They will gather together thousands of other like-minded people into an organization called Birthright, the alternative to abortion.

Meanwhile, another woman from Kansas is flying to the same destinations, Minneapolis, with a similar mission in mind: to meet with a woman who has a plan for direct action to aid women distressed by pregnancy. Her name is Bernadette Sanders.

A few months later a mother of four is preparing a special soup to be served to her pastor in the hopes of obtaining his financial assistance to fund a group known as Birthright in her city of Richland, Washington. M.T. Hall.

In Missoula, Montana a mother passes the time with her 3-month old infant by watching the Phil Donahue show on TV. He is interviewing a guest from Right To Life. The guest tells of the work of a group called Birthright. She sends for a copy of The *Story of Birthright* and opens an office with others in her city. Nancy Morton.

In Eugene, Oregon, a mother of five is reading her diocesan newspaper. She is drawn to an article on a new pro-life group in Portland, Oregon.

She calls the Director. They meet and an office is opened in March of 1973 in Eugene.

In California, Paula Vandegaer, a Sister of Social Work, hears the news that a bill allowing abortion has passed. She, too, has met Louise Summerhill and Sister Paula wonders how she can help. Sister calls five colleagues together. They write a manual to help guide lay people in their work with distressed pregnant women.

When we follow the stories of these women we find that they fulfilled their dreams to push back against the abortion behemoth by creating and participating in a movement. It has come to be called the Pro-Life Service Movement.

Louise Summerhill is the woman that these people had come to depend upon to fight abortion. Her idea of providing practical help to every woman distressed by an unplanned pregnancy is key. When Louise became aware that there was a 24-hour hotline which provided Canadian women with places in New York State for abortions, she decided to found a hotline but a saving one with the added feature of an office staffed by caring, knowledgeable people--all volunteers--who would offer help to carry the baby to term with dignity and peace.

I am not the first to speak of the history of the movement. In addition to Louise's own book, *The Story of Birthright* (Summerhill, 1968), others have already begun to tell the story from their various perspectives. Some of these have been less than favorable and have even characterized the pro-life outreach of Crisis Pregnancy Centers as places using scare tactics on desperate and unsuspecting women. For example, CPC's are said to force women to watch videos or as second rate places where volunteers dole out infant formula and hand-me-down clothing. I can say in all honesty that this last statement does not describe any CPC's with which I am personally aware.

Seeing that others have already begun to tell the story of this grassroots movement, I have been moved to share my personal experience of how the movement has evolved from its beginning. As of the writing of this book there are basically two models of CPC's though these are run by many various groups. The approach used by 1st Way has as its goal saving innocent lives from abortion so that these precious human beings can someday hear the gospel. I believe that this was the original vision of CPCs. Therefore, it should not be a requirement to apply any pressure to our client to accept faith. Nor is it wise, in my opinion to encourage a reputation that clients will be encouraged to accept religion by pro-lifers in general. While some clients may be reached by this other method, which is a faith based approach that actively tries to bring the mother to faith, it will not work for everyone and may cause them to avoid our assistance completely. Since our first priority is saving all unborn babies from abortion we must focus on basic needs with all our strength. Ultimately, however, both the neutral approach and the faith-based approach have a unity of goals, which is to protect the unborn and their mothers.

The difference in method does sometimes lead to a greater disunity in the movement. As I will discuss, pro-lifers are very independent folks and we have sometimes found ourselves competing for volunteers and funding instead of cooperating. Passions can run very deep in support of one method or the other and for some the difference can not be set aside. Both the original neutral approach and the faith-based model have had successes worth noting in saving unborn lives. It is my hope that competitive attitudes will fade altogether through mutual understanding and that we can celebrate and support our mutual goals. Patrick J. Riley wrote a book review of *Habits of Compassion* (Fitzgerald, 2006) which is relevant both to the CPCs of modern times and to my purpose in writing this book. Riley reinforces the rightness of nurturing intuition in Habits which chronicles the efforts of religious sisters in the United States in creating and sustaining Catholic schools, hospitals and institutions and programs of social welfare. Riley identifies such compassionate endeavors as a subcategory of women's history and a rich one that needs to be told in its many manifestations. The story of Crisis Pregnancy Centers (CPC), our story, that emerged from 1968 on into the 21st Century falls into this manifestation of rich history. It is a direct result and expression of the drive and the vision on the part of ordinary women with nurturing intuition who have stepped up to combat abortion face to face and to help pregnant women to live in peace.

There is a quote from Flannery O'Connor's work I would like to suggest succinctly describes workers at the CPC: "We have the unsentimental eye of acceptance which is to say, faith" (O'Connor, 2008). There is no room for whitewashing or emotionalism on the front lines of the battle against abortion. Faith must be the thing that sustains us in the face of this evil. Faith that one is called to the work. Faith that God is good and the battle is worth fighting.

The founding of Birthright and the founding of our own center in Eugene, Oregon as well as hundreds of others across the country have been the first responders meeting an urgent need. My experience from the very beginning of these crisis centers has been one guided by love. Though it has also been filled with difficult personal and financial struggles, it has yielded fruit with value beyond measure, which is human life itself. This book is the story of our labor. It is a work of love.

CHAPTER 1.

The Abortion Challenge: What We Were Up Against

The abortion milieu was prepared by academics. On the national stage people who considered themselves part of an elite, eugenicists, who fervently believed there were too many people on earth, were in the forefront. They were writers, activists like Margaret Sanger (Drogin, 1979), Charles Devenport, Sir Francis Galton, and sociologists like Havelock Ellis (Ellis, 1911) and Henry Fairchild (Fairchild, 1977).

Closer to home in Eugene at the U of O professors were stressing the coming doom due to human births gone wild, for example, Paul Erlich's *The Population Bomb* (1968).

Meanwhile, paradoxically, the federal and state governments introduced grants for the poor so that they became dependent on the government for help.

Gone were the days when middle and upper class women from the private sector led their contemporaries into movements to protect children from dire economic straits on their own resources, like Helen Hull and her Hull House. Institutions such as orphanages which saved children from the street and work houses, chronicled in books like *Habits of Compassion* (Fitzgerald, 2006), were, by the 60's, looked upon with loathing. Even adoption came under suspicion. A new characteristic was emerging for the pregnant woman. She would be autonomous but funded by the welfare state.

Welfare rights movements of the 1950s and 1960s which stressed equality of opportunity, especially in education, received political affirmation from the top. Presidents Kennedy, Johnson, Carter, and Clinton all said that society was to be organized to help the poor through programs like Aid to Dependent Children.

Ideals of the great society proposed and pushed initially by intellectuals and then by government were to provide pathways using legislative means to enable segments of American society to get ahead. The stated intent was more and better jobs, especially for women. The 1990s Welfare to Work movement was a later development, yet the entire system severely weakened the two parent family concept. The mother was to be a worker outside of the home, causing even greater demands for child care.

What happened instead of the Great Society, from my vantage point, was that the idea of the family wage, where the father provided for his wife and children, was lost. By 1971 public welfare became a federal government domain, with a budget in 1972 of 1.7 billion. It grew each year and included payment for abortion.

At our office in Eugene, Title XX eligibility standards provided single pregnant women with social services like rent for an apartment, food stamps, Aid to Dependent Children, WIC, etc. Although fewer funds in Oregon were available, it seemed to us money was always found for abortions. In addition, Oregon had fewer restrictions for residence so many needy women settled here. The "absent father rule" which said benefits were restricted to those who disclosed the name of the father were overlooked and aid was provided nevertheless.

In the decades of the 70's and 80's America, and from my perspective, Eugene was suffering from a sort of schizophrenia. On the one hand, Feminism with its relentless demand for more recognition, power, and prestige for women would portray the traditional role of motherhood as a "second slavery," being continuously characterized by such writers as Germaine Greer and Gloria Steinam. On the other hand, the back to the land movement with the birth of a baby as a key element, was immortalized by the writings of Ina Mae Gaskin

(1975) in her book, *Spiritual Midwifery*. It became a vision to be followed by a certain segment of Oregon's childbearing population. Even OB specialists like Dr. Mayer Eisentein proclaimed the "home court advantage." Ironically, in spite of the best efforts of hospitals to attract clients to their "birthing rooms" by making the hospital look more like home, the stress of malpractice suits on OB doctors were forcing many to give up delivering babies altogether. Some doctors would not accept welfare patients.

In 1973 the Supreme Court handed down two infamous decisions, Roe and Bolton. These decisions allowed and then fostered abortion on demand for all nine months of pregnancy, overturning most states laws and unleashing a true holocaust on the unborn. In the next two years, for example, South Carolina's judicial decision provided a respected venue upon which abortionists could perform the procedure. These precedents spread to all states. Abortionists could then advertize and establish clinics.[1]

More court decisions even allowed non-physicians to perform the abortion. After Biglow v Va, Connecticut v Nenilla in 1975 and Singleton v Wiliff abortionists could receive state and federal reimbursement for their services.[2] In 1976 Planned Parenthood of Central Mass v Danforth won a victory against the family. The court rejected parental involvement in the abortion decision of their minor child. Even the fathers were denied rights over their unborn children. States could fund abortions and even saline abortions were permitted. These were indeed performed at OHS in Portland. In Eugene, All Women's Health Center was established in 1984 and performed abortions up to 22 weeks. Now Bours clinic has taken its place.

The Christian Medical Association of Oregon was very careful not to anger their abortion colleagues. Yet the International Federation of Prolife Doctors was evidence that many doctors were not comfortable with the addition of abortion to their skills and duties.

---

[1] National Right to Life Committee "1998 Yearbook." Edited by Lisa Andrusco.
[2] National Right to Life Educational Trust Fund, "Supreme Court Decisions."

On the local scene, as soon as Roe became law, most OB/GYNs gave in and performed abortions in their offices or in the local hospital but after 10 years only a few remained providers. It is not a procedure for the faint of heart and additionally a stigma has grown against performing abortions in OB/GYN offices. Doctors are used to working on life issues, therefore abortion was left to hard core doctors working in freestanding clinics like the Lovejoy Clinic in Portland and Bours clinic in Eugene and Forest Grove. The attitudes of these hard core doctors may be similar to that of Dr. Bernard Nathanson (1981), who, before his conversion, thought that his abortion work was helping to prevent infections in women who tried to self abort.

In addition, there was a difficulty for our clients over welfare payments for hospital delivery. The Oregon Health Plan did not include women with some financial resources, a percentage of women with incomes over the poverty line were denied access to care. Also, in the 1980s I remember a big push by welfare workers to have girls take the Depo Provera shot. At the office, we heard about the unpleasant effects from clients. I myself, when I accompanied a pregnant girl to her appointment with her caseworker, heard the worker say, "After your baby you should get on the Depo Provera shot or Norplant." Many of these services, especially the Oregon Health Plan, have been expanded, but birth control is still strongly encouraged.

I knew that the following kind of conversation went on with many of our clients anytime they applied for welfare payments, even in the hospital just after birth, the question was asked by the nurse: So, what kind of birth control will you be using? The pill? It was standard and many of the girls caved into this pressure. It was embarrassing for them to decline the help since they were getting free delivery on the State, as it were.

The year 1980 was a peak year for abortions. It was disappointing that in 1981 the Hatch amendment to the Constitution was defeated. It would have outlawed abortions with exceptions of those caused by rape/incest. It was defeated by a pro-life group which demanded no exceptions.

The entire realm of services for pregnant women has become filled with dilemmas for doctors, particularly those with strong personal views respecting life. How could they reconcile their belief with their patient's desires?

There had not been much growth in cooperation between the Eugene crisis pregnancy centers and doctors. In 1998 the Board suggested we develop a program of outreach to local doctors. A questionnaire was devised. We called at 18 local doctors offices to describe our services. (For example, a volunteer did 40 loads of wash at home, another cleaned her house.) A few doctors granted personal interviews and we found two doctors supportive. The rest remained aloof. On the other hand, two stalwart OB groups have ventured to stand with us. One is our Medical Director.

Finding shelter homes is an essential need for many of our clients but it became more difficult to find after the Gerard House, a residential care facility for pregnant women closed around 1976. By 1985 a new home, Orchard Inn, which was run by a Christian group, came into being. We sent lots of our clients there, but that too closed after eleven years because of personnel problems.

Through the years, our girls were changing as well. In the past we could go with them to the hospital because they were essentially alone but now more and more friends or moms and boyfriends attended births. The stigma of unwed birth has dramatically declined, although some girls still face birth alone and we are still there for them; there is still a need for proper housing for them.

In early 1991 the local Planned Parenthood attempted, as a member of Lane County Teen Pregnancy Task Force, to get the other members of the group to prohibit Birthright, also a member, from advertising in high school newspapers. I engaged a lawyer, Tom Alderman, to write a letter threatening suit if they pursued their plan to forbid access of BR to school papers. Planned Parenthood withdrew its request.

School-based clinics were set up in 1993. By 1997, every high school in Eugene had one. These clinics, while claiming to take care of students who were sick, also included pregnancy testing in their services.

In general, CPCs do not involve themselves in the political side of the abortion issue. Our service is to mothers directly and already requires all of the time, effort and financial resources that we have. Nonetheless, political issues sometimes come to us or are simply too big to ignore for the impact that they have upon our work. There have been some legal assaults from groups such as NARAL, which we have been forced to respond to in order to keep our doors open, such as a pamphlet entitled "The Choice Action Kit: A Step by Step guide to Unmasking Fake Clinics." In the late 1990s, claims were made that CPCs used fear tactics. Bills supported by Eliot Spitzer (then New York Attorney General) in 2002 and a bill in 2006 sponsored by Representative Maloney of NY sought to investigate pro-life centers for inappropriate practices. Here in Oregon, SB776 was defeated in 2007 but will return in another form. We are grateful for the support of interested citizens who believe in the need for pro-life centers in beating back these attempts by petitioning their legislatures. One reason we are able to keep informed is the assistance of organizations such at Right to Life. The *RTL News* has helped inform us of these legislative attacks. We are joyful when we hear that 76% of Americans are against abortion, but we know that the political battle is deeper than any one poll.

On the flip side, there also have been many success in legislation to protect women, for example, parental notification laws. There have been some attempts by legislatures to help pregnancy centers. For example, the Pregnant and Parenting Student Services Act of 2005 advocated using colleges to provide services to pregnant and parenting students on their campuses. Sadly this measure has not been enacted. The Born Alive Infants Protection Act of 2006 also has not been enacted.

Once, holding aloof from advertising the good of adoption in public schools, adoption agencies have used federal grants to conduct inservice training to educate crisis pregnancy volunteers on how to present adoption in more appealing ways.

Nonetheless due to the Supreme Court decision in Casey vs. Planned Parenthood (1992) our society continued to growing more and more schizophrenic, wanting autonomy by violent means. Abortion is viewed by some people as dirty, an unpleasant part of life and a private matter. As Justice Kennedy said, "We, as society have become dependent on abortion."

I do not agree that we are dependent upon it, but abortion has certainly become ingrained in our culture. Now there is even Internet access directly to abortionists. Yet the challenge to abortion as status quo remains. Possiblypregnant.org, our own website shows that the voice of dissent, of love, and of the true support for human life remains active in our culture as well.

CHAPTER 2.

Prolife Influences:
The People We Depended On

The year 1973 was marked by horrendous sorrow and shocking wakeup call to many, because of Roe. However, the years running up to the fateful decisions Roe and Bolton were not sleepy nor indolent years for everyone. Abortion on demand and its effects were known to some. They sought to motivate the public to support prolife efforts.

There were many people and events which have shaped our culture, specifically in regards to abortion, since I joined the CPC movement. I can give only a sampling of these but would like to share some of those that had greatest impact upon the CPCs, especially, our center in Eugene, OR. Of course there are many others examples and individuals which may even have had broader influence. My goal is only to share those that were the most apparent and significant from my own perspective in the field.

Father Paul Marx was a leader in the pro-life movement in the early 1970s. He was prescient in seeing that abortion would soon follow contraception. His many books and pamphlets were essential resources to us in the early years. He called upon the nobility of men to acknowledge and respond to their innate responsibility to women and children. His advice was always very practical without demeaning women at all.

Following Fr. Marx, was Dr. Eugene Diamond of Chicago, an OB doctor and charter member of the International Federation of

Prolife Doctors. To my knowledge not one doctor in Eugene became a member. The Christian Medical Association of Oregon was very careful to avoid any public announcements regarding the practice of abortion. In fact, many doctors engaged in the abortion procedure from 1973 until the mid 80's.

By the late 80's the procedure was limited to a few hardcore physicians. In Oregon they practiced in free standing clinics like Lovejoy and Bours.

The next hero was Dr. Bernard Nathanson, an abortionist with over 60,000 abortions on his record. A stalwart member of NARAL, he testifies in his book, *Aborting America,* that he colluded with NARAL when testifying before Congress, to inflate the number of illegal abortions prior to Roe to one million when statistics proved to be an infinitesimal amount less. His conversion story is one of inspiration and thankfulness to the grace of God. Dr. Thomas Hilgers and Dr. John Horan, who wrote *Abortion and Social Justice,* were enlightening as well.

Another hero is Henry Hyde who managed to shepherd in 1976 the amendment to Congress that prevented the Federal Government from paying for abortions. His great work has lasted until the present when President Obama reversed the Mexico City policy by executive order so that taxpayers now pay for abortions at home and abroad.

Dr. John Wilke, an OB from Ohio, took his place along side the other prolife pioneers by writing and lecturing on the evils of abortion. His *Handbook on Abortion* (Wilke, 1971) became a sort of bible for the pregnancy centers. He wrote clearly and authoritatively on the various abortions procedures with an eye to helping lay people to understand what abortion was and thus help the pregnant woman and her baby. His influence in promoting prolife activities is still felt today especially in legislative venues.

The pioneer for urging participation in prolife causes, especially the CPC's, was Fr. John Powell. He rightly described abortion as the new

"Holocaust" on the vulnerable unborn. His early books and lectures inspired prolife workers to begin the fight.

Fr. Frank Pavone, founder of Priests for Life, has written, lectured and produced radio and TV programs that continually challenge and inform listeners on the duties of all citizens to use their talents to defend life.

Dr. James Dobson, another pioneer in the prolife movement, used his considerable talents to found an organization called "Focus on the Family." His radio broadcast over 30 years have served to inspire and inform lay people to defend the unborn. He is still a powerful voice in the fight for life.

Nancy Jo Mann, a victim of abortion herself, founded an organization called "Women Exploited by Abortion." Other women traveled the United States giving testimony to the horrendous effects of abortion on their own lives. Her group was a very valuable resource for training of our volunteers.

The inspired action of Joe Schiedler, who early in the abortion wars, decided to meet and talk with pregnant women at the site of the killing fields, the abortion clinics themselves, was another approach. His approach is called "sidewalk counseling."

Monsignor Phillip Reilly, originator and still active participant in the life saving movement called "God's Precious Innocents" has inspired many others to engage in sidewalk counseling. This has been a good team effort for our centers because sometimes they bring women to our clinics.

I could not conclude without praising the efforts of one lone woman, Marian Banducci of California. She continues to educate young people on the evils of abortion with her pamphleteering at high schools in California. Her book, *20 Years on the Front Lines*, is a tribute to perseverance with grace (Banducci, 2003).

Another group called "Operation Rescue" captured headlines and television coverage with its radical approach. Its members would chain themselves to the abortion clinic venues. They suffered abuse from police and served jail and prison time for their actions. The courts finally stopped these activities when the leader, Randall Terry, was condemned and fined for his leadership.

Joan Andrews was one valiant woman who spent precious years of her life in federal prison for her silent defense of the unborn at abortion clinics. She was one of the first to suffer such punishment as part of the government plan to severely curtail the civil rights of prolifers.

From 1970 to 1980 many other groups with prolife agendas blossomed and grew. There was the Right to Life organization of the late 60's, the Right to Life Committee formed in May of 1973. There were political action groups at all of the state levels. The American Life League was founded by Judie Brown in 1984 and the March for Life was formed by Nellie Gray in 1974. It continues to gather huge crowds in Washington, DC, on January 22, commemorating the Roe decision.

Some prolifers have taken an investigative approach like Mark Crutcher (1996) of Denton, Texas. Working with undercover people he wrote about abortionists who sell baby parts and detailed their grizzly actions in his book, *Lime 5: Exploited by Choice.*

The medical community can be proud of one famous member, Dr. Jerome Lejeune[3] of Paris, who has written much on the wonder of life.

From 1970 to 1984 the Catholic Church, through the Bishops, was one of the only voices in public opposition to abortion. The Church was roundly criticized and ridiculed for her stance and there was little alliance or support from any other group for more than a decade.

---

[3] Tennessee Circuit Court for Blount Co. Davis v King, Seven Frozen Embryos. Case No E-14496, 1989. Blount Co, Tennessee.

Curtis Young entered the movement around 1984 and founded the Christian Action Council and its many groups, which are now known under the umbrella name "CareNet" (Koop & Schaefer, 1983). These groups are composed of dedicated Evangelicals (Ensor, 2003) and are well funded by their church mission boards. They offer help as CPCs do and generally follow the same prolife program but added the component of proselytizing to their program.

New programs to help post-abortion women, such as Rachel's Vineyard, were inspired by Dr. Theresa Burke. *Silent No More Campaign,* instituted by Fr. Pavone and Janet Marana is another important development.

Even Hollywood has made popular movies about adoption like "Bella" and "Juno."

CHAPTER 3.

Personal Stories

Directors and volunteers at eight different centers have shared with me some of their stories. I want to share them here so that you can see the similarities among many clinics across the United States. The grassroots beginnings of each of these crisis pregnancy centers are similar to our own in Eugene. Also, the drive to serve pregnant women in their time of need is expressed by these women much as it has been felt by myself and the volunteers I have worked with. These workers are also volunteers, sharing the struggle to balance their own families with the urgent need to combat the evil of abortion by meeting each pregnant woman face to face in friendship.

<ins>Oregon</ins>

Lucy Berg, a veteran volunteer of 35 years at our own Eugene Birthright/1st Way shares the following.

When Roe became the law, pro-life people began to realize that something had to be done to combat abortion. The Birthright group was the answer for me. The charter would keep us focused. The mission, to give pregnant women a positive help and reassurance, was what I was looking for. At the meeting I saw that funds were donated and an office was rented. It was in an old building. We were all learning but all were dedicated to helping clients and wanted to save precious lives.

One inspiring event for me was the conference at the University of Notre Dame where I met pro-life people from all over the USA. The idea of leaving a better world for our grandchildren keeps me coming for my shift week after week.

I feel that maybe these pregnant women have no one else that prays for them so after they leave I pray for them. I have never wanted to quit or been afraid in this movement because I believe in following through on my commitments. I am happy because I've learned a lot and met wonderful volunteers. I believe in the basic goodness of our fellow human beings. We are all God's children and some of us are just luckier to be born into good families that teach us about God's plan. I am hopeful in the technology of the ultrasound.

Kansas

By far the most complete contribution I have received came from Bernadette Sanders in Wichita, Kansas, so it is her stories that I would like to share first. The following history of their center is largely in her own words, though edited and paraphrased where appropriate for presentation in this book.

I attended the Right to Life meeting in Minnesota where Louise Summerhill presented her idea of Birthright, a crisis pregnancy center. Later in August 1971 I was invited by Louise to attend a meeting to finalize the Birthright Charter. The most challenging innovation of the Birthright centers was that lay people, non-professionals would do the counseling of girls and women in crisis.

In the early years Birthright International was very vigilant to protect the Charter, using legal action if necessary for violations. Louise knew that if the Birthright Charter was not protected, there would be no Birthright. Every center would operate as they pleased. Incredibly there were even some centers that referred for abortion in certain cases. It seemed that almost at every convention we had Gordon Kaiser, trademark lawyer, speak about the Birthright logo, the "B" with the phone inside, and the vision of the Charter. There were some other lawsuits by Birthright? One against a company wanting to market creams and lotions to pregnant women. They called themselves "Birthright." Our Birthright successfully was able to stop them. However, this cost Birthright International lots of money and centers were asked to help with this.

Locally we experienced camping out at our center by lawyers seeking to get babies from our clients. They actually approached women outside our center and others and offered large sums of money if the client would place her baby for adoption. Birthright International acted quickly to forbid all private adoptions at BR centers.

Another restriction was our inability to refer our clients for Natural Family Planning, a purely natural method of spacing children. Because we were interdenominational, we were told it was to be treated as just another method of birth control.

Birthright International was able to monitor its centers in part through the Regional Consultants. Ideally each state would have one, though the smaller states often shared one. I became a consultant for Kansas. As Regional Consultant it was my responsibility to see to it that the Charter was being followed exactly. For more than 20 years Kansas and Oklahoma centers, Regional Consultants decided to combine annual meetings for directors and office managers. It was a way of maintaining contact and helping these centers through their Directors. During this time my husband, a CP, provided help with incorporation along with my training for approximately 20 centers in Kansas. This continued until the early 1990"s.

After Louise died and the three daughters took over, it seemed many things changed at Birthright International. One of the Summerhill twins is a lawyer and perhaps that is where the following new rule came from. In Canada's political system not only was abortion legal, but if you speak against it, you can be considered anti-government. Therefore, Birthrights were not allowed to speak against abortion. This seems to me a contradiction to the position held by Louise all the years I knew her. In 1994 our BR changed its name to Birthline.

Wichita Birthline is among the most active pregnancy centers performing over 1,000 pregnancy tests. An ultrasound machine on the premises is not thought to be necessary as the Birthline clients have access to a nearby hospital clinic, which provides and performs free ultrasounds for their women. Incredible, inspiring stories follow.

In the early years, when I received Louise's manuscript, *The Story of Birthright* (Summerhill, 1968), several of us felt it was something we could and should do. I still felt like Louise used to say, "Dear Lord surely you can find someone more suitable to lead this movement." With the encouragement of my husband Bill and prayer I knew it would fall on me if it were to go forward. I was fortunate to have a nun, Sister Madeline, whom I knew through Lamaze classes, that was also very interested in getting Birthright started. She would write sketchy minutes of the early meetings, who was there, and a next plan of action. After she typed them we could send them to interested persons. This was the beginning of our current newsletters. By the way, Sister Madeleine was years later named to the International Birthright Board of Directors. Fr. Reinhard Eck, Our pastor in 1971, has always been available with his wise counsel getting started and through all these years. He is currently a board member.

We continued to have meetings and our enthusiasm increased especially when Fr. Larson, Director of Catholic Charities, allowed us the use of a room in an unused convent. We always said that the pregnancy test was our trump card in that it was what brought the girls to us. Thinking back to those early tests. Wow! We had to mix drops of urine with drops of solution on a glass slide. If the result was grainy, the test was negative. If it was smooth as milk (it was white), it was positive. We have sure come a long way in that regard.

In our first five years I think we moved 4 times always relying on generous businessmen giving us free rent. Our movers (husbands) were getting weary of the moves so we looked for a house to buy. There was a trend across the country in that direction. I contacted a local realtor, someone I knew from grade school and high school, and asked if he knew of a house. He personally owned this house. In fact, a family was living in it. After he verbally told me a price he later asked me to repeat it so he could write it down because he wouldn't believe it otherwise. It was as though an angel whispered in his ear,

"They really need this property." We have been in this house for 31 years. He had purchased it for its ideal commercial location. It was, and still is, the ideal location for us.

Bill and I and Sister Madeleine traveled to the first international conventions and later on a number of our volunteers joined us. In alternating years the conventions were in the US and Canada. We met so many wonderful people from the US and Canada and really felt a part of a very large picture. We always felt energized after attending these meetings.

After we were open for 5 years I became pregnant. We were thrilled after waiting and praying for 9 years for another child. I asked Denise, the National Birthright Director about the possibility of resigning. She suggested that I consider naming an Office Manager, which I did. Diane Bebak became Office Manager and from that time on we became a team. So much so that my mother said Diane and I were as close as sisters. We consulted with each other on most of the decisions relating to our center.

The timing of all of this was perfect because around that same time I was named by Denise and Louise to be Regional Consultant for the State of Kansas. If anyone in Kansas was interested in more information on Birthright, perhaps starting a center in their community my name was given to them. In the years to follow Bill and I traveled to many cities in Kansas and provided training for an additional 19 centers. I was available to them by phone for any questions regarding their center.

I encouraged all of them, especially the Directors, to attend the International Conventions and then at some time during the Convention all Kansas delegated met. These were wonderful times. Times of building friendships while honing our skills for the important work we had all committed to. In later years Barbara Chishko, Director of BR of Oklahoma City, and Diane and I planned and held Regional Director meetings annually in Oklahoma City and Wichita alternately for the Directors and key people of the centers in Oklahoma and Kansas. Wichita BR purchased all the many brochures in bulk and then we were able to sell to each of the centers at a reduced rate.

The role of the Director of a center is simply to keep things going. Specifically maintaining adequate and competent staff (all volunteers), raising monies to cover all expenses and most importantly getting out the message that you exist so girls and women who need your services know how and where to reach you. Advertising has always been one of our biggest expenses. I always felt that it was very important to maintain a positive image in the community without compromising our pro-life position.

I felt fortunate that we never had to do fund raising. Because no salaries were ever paid in 36 years our expenses were dramatically less than many other centers. I have always heard that a major part of the budget of many a charitable non-profit organization is often salaries. At board meetings when we presented statistics of the numbers of people served the previous year, the attorney on our board was always amazed at the number of people served with such a small amount of money. Our quarterly newsletter brings in the money we need to operate. In each newsletter we include a return envelope. This works great.

In 1971 when we began much was made of the fact that New York State had the most liberal abortion law in the country with abortions being allowed until the 24th week. Much was being made of when viability of the baby was present. The truth of those times was that Kansas had no time limit on abortion. We have for all these years had an abortionist in Wichita who is known nationally as a late-term abortionist. We at Birthline have interviewed a number of girls and women from Minnesota, North Caroline, etc. who came to Wichita for abortions after 6 months of pregnancy. The culture of death has only progressed in all of these years. I believe the media, TV and the movie industry played a huge role in this. However, I believe that the decrease in the number of pregnancies and abortions is a direct result of the pro-life movement. The hundreds of crisis pregnancy centers, I believe, deserve much of the credit for this decline.

We have a long way to go to be considered a "culture of life." When a middle school decides it needs to provide contraceptives to its students without parents' knowledge, something is terribly wrong with our culture's ability to solve problems.

The fact that God didn't send Bill and I the large family (we had three children) that my brothers and sisters had, allowed us to do all of the traveling needed during the formation of all the new centers and the annual conventions. Bill's parents helped us a lot in that area. While money was never a big issue in Wichita, maintaining a volunteer staff to cover 6 days a week was indeed a challenge. Currently we have a staff of 30 volunteers. Another challenge is getting those volunteers to attend "mandatory" volunteer meetings every 2 months. We initially had them every month but changed to bi-monthly to accommodate our volunteers. I believe it is so important to keep everyone on the same page regarding policies, current issues and on-going training in answering abortion calls and counseling walk-in clients. We have been blessed with a very high caliber of volunteer with very little turnover. Because so many organizations are asking for volunteers, it seems more difficult to recruit new volunteers. I also find that it seems more and more people are less willing to make commitments.

Offering the option of adoption to a girl or woman continues to be a real challenge. In the current culture it seems placing a baby for adoption is so foreign to most of the women we see. They almost seem insulted that it is even offered. If she is a young teen, her mother usually responds with something like: "Oh, no, we will raise the baby. We love babies." Statistically girls over 20 are more apt to place their babies than those under 20.

Counseling at our center seems to have changed a lot from the early years. It was easier to reach an abortion minded woman then. The abortion mentality is so ingrained in our culture today that even someone with a religious background will more easily rationalize an abortion. There was a time when we believed that making the baby real to her seemed to make a difference. Showing her the baby models, brochures, etc. but today it seems that she is more concerned about herself and what the baby will do to her life.

Wichita has three crisis pregnancy centers. One of them is located in an area that serves much of the African American population. Birthline serves much of the Hispanic community. The language barrier does present its problems. We have a series of cards that what might be considered a list of needs she might have, translated in Spanish. This seems to work well for us. Beyond this we have interpreters we can call.

We are fortunate in Wichita to have available to us an organization/ medical clinic: Choices Medical Clinic. They will provide a 4D sonogram for our abortion minded women and girls. They exist primarily for the purpose of providing ultrasound technology to abortion minded women in the Wichita and surrounding communities. While many crisis pregnancy centers now provide this service, we see no reason to provide it since we are able to use Choice Medical Clinic. Not all girls will agree to go there but those who do seem to have a favorable outcome.

I'm reminded of a young woman who came to Birthline seeking an abortion. Our volunteers convinced her to go to Choices for a sonogram. She carried the baby to term. A year and a half later she returned with a beautiful little girl who was in her words "the love of my life." Yet unbelievably, she was again thinking of abortion.

The person who was most influential in me getting involved and staying involved was my husband, Bill. He was and is totally supportive, provides a great sounding board. I could always bounce ideas off of him and, of course, he traveled with me. No one knows the many behind the scenes projects or odd jobs he has willingly provided for our center.

My future dreams are simple: that the work of Birthline in Wichita will continue.

Case History – Angie

Angie walked into *Birthline* one Saturday morning in July. She had called earlier in the week saying she needed to talk to someone. She was from Western Kansas and was told we were open Saturday 10-1.

She dropped in the chair and began crying so much she couldn't speak. When she finally composed herself, she was "all over the page" – very emotionally distraught. I let her talk as long as she wished and then repeated back to her what I heard her say to make sure I understood the facts and the emotions.

She spilled out her predicament: She has an eight year old son with serious medical problems. His father left when Andy was a baby. Angie has watched Andy struggle, having no father, and vowed she would not do that to another child … And here she was eight weeks pregnant!! The current boyfriend walked out saying "marriage is out of the question." He said he didn't care what she did, but when she mentioned adoption he blew up. Saying he would "never give permission and I'll fight for custody". I still pursued the adoption possibility, but she was adamant that she couldn't give up the baby after carrying for nine months. Even so, I went over the adoption questionnaire as it helped sort out feeling and other important factors. When we came to the other options she had considered – the only one was abortion.

I explained that would be a quick fix, but a decision she would live with the rest of her life. I showed her the exact replica model of a baby as approximately her baby's age and asked if she would consider meeting with a social worker from Catholic Social Services, as they offer pregnancy counseling. "Well, maybe," she replied.

I told her I would get in touch with an attorney who has been very helpful to *Birthline* and ask about some legal concerns she had: and also with Catholic Social Services to find a counselor in Western Kansas, near her home.

I asked if she had picked out a name for the baby. "Yes, Seth." I said, "Angie, you have already bonded with your baby, haven't you?" She began to cry again. I told her I could tell she really didn't want to destroy the baby.

Birthline was closing, so I asked if I could take her to lunch. She agreed and we talked until 3:30. When she left, she had decided to carry her baby and would like advice from our attorney and also Catholic Social Services.

After talking with the attorney and locating a social worker in Western Kansas, I called Angie on Wednesday with the information. She responded saying that we were just what she needed at the time; people who would listen to her and really care. She said she hadn't cried since Saturday.

She also said she had called *Birthline* after hours and heard our 2 minute message and called back 3 times to listen again. Angie's baby is due in spring!!

Anna's Story

Sometime in the Spring of 2006, a young girl came to *Birthline* for a test. Ironically, she came on the same day of the week with the same volunteers she had talked to 1 ½ years ago when she was 17 years old. The volunteer recognized her and remembered her as having come for a Positive test and then asking for an abortion.

Eighteen months ago Anna (not her real name) was living with her father and sisters. Their mother had died and they had immigrated to this country. Anna was very talented in sports and was counting on a college scholarship. A pregnancy did not fit in the picture, so an abortion seemed the only solution.

Our volunteers had arranged for her to obtain a free sonogram. We know that often when a mother can see her baby, she is less apt to destroy it. This was the last contact with Anna. All we could do was pray.

Now, fast forward 1 ½ years and again Anna is in for a test. She has with her a beautiful one year old daughter she refers to as "my best friend". Again the results of the test are Positive. Unbelievably, again she wants an abortion.

When the possibility of adoption is presented to her, she is receptive. An appointment is made for her with Catholic Charities but it was learned later that she did not keep this appointment.

Attempts to reach her have been unsuccessful. It is believed that she shares a cell phone with her sisters.

We **pray** that God will protect Anna and her baby as he did 1 ½ years ago.

Washington

This story from the Birthright serving Spokane and Richland was contributed by M. T. Hall, past Director of the Birthright center. Her story echoes the personal investment of other centers. Hope, gratitude, and humility are the mainstays of her approach to the challenge of helping mothers and children.

About 30 years ago my friend invited me to a meeting of women who were thinking about organizing a pregnancy aid service. At the time of the meeting, I was pregnant again and turned down the job of Treasurer, but said I was definitely interested in volunteering. I myself had a child out of wedlock when I was 22 and my parents had coerced me into placing him for adoption. My sympathies were in place. Interestingly enough it took 9 months until our center was ready to open. By that time, the gal who had been our director was leaving town. She said that we never would have gotten as far as we did, except for my calling her, almost daily, with ideas for what we needed to do. The result is that I ended up as the director of our Birthright. By the time we opened, I had a two-month-old baby myself.

One of the first women who came to our center was so delighted to be pregnant I was moved to give her a blanket. I myself, then a mother of four, had never been given a baby shower. The woman was happy and as she was going out the door said, "My husband will be so happy." Then she started tearing, stepped back inside and told me her story. This was her fourth pregnancy but would be their third baby. When she was last pregnant, she had gone to Planned Parenthood.

Her husband was unemployed at the time, and the woman there put a huge guilt trip on her. The woman was very negative regarding when her husband might be employed again. She told her that she had no business putting further burden on her husband, it wasn't fair to the children she already had, etc. The worst was that the woman convinced her to have an abortion without consulting her husband! When he later found out what she had done, he was crushed. He said, "Do you really have so little faith in me that you thought I wouldn't take care of my family?" She said he was so angry; it was only by God's grace that their marriage survived at all. Her visit to our center in its earliest days was confirmation that we were as needed as we had thought.

Even an all-volunteer group needs some money. We had none. I was not by nature inclined to ask people for money but I new we had to. I called the pastor of my parish and invited him to have lunch with me and the gal who was our director at the time. I made African chicken peanut soup. While we dined, we told him about our venture. He immediately wrote a check for $2,000. I still think of my African chicken peanut soup as my $2,000 Plate dinner recipe.

Our first office was upstairs, down a long dark hall, in an old building. It was far from ideal, but perhaps it felt OK to the girls who were so desperate they may have in fact though we were going to help them obtain an abortion. Since I had a tiny baby, as did other volunteers, we were not inclined to spend more than one day a week in the office. I took care of children for another volunteer and she took care of mine on the days we worked.

I had gone to pro-life conferences on a couple of occasions. Just prior to opening our Birthright, I attended a Birthright conference in Oregon. This is where I met Terry Ianora and Denise Cocciolone. After that, I attended many Birthright conferences. I was fortunate in that our Birthright provided for me to attend. I really loved the conferences and always felt a bit guilty that more volunteers weren't able to attend. The Birthright Charter was the first I had heard of. I have not studied the charters of other pregnancy aid centers in detail.

Even so, I think that limiting our focus is the right thing to do. Our centers cannot be all things to all people. It is easier to continue to do well if we do not overtax the time and energy of our volunteers. It is also easier to control the experience of the clients if we do not have volunteers trying to do too much, e.g., proselytize, solve fertility problems, etc.

I think the most important virtue a person must have in order to do the work is humility. If we had good parents, upbringing, or education, it was a gift from God. If we had a terrible life, it may help us in relating and assisting the women who come to us. In any case, we cannot credit ourselves when we are able to point a girl in the right direction. Any good that happens is done through us but hardly ever by us. No headway can ever be made unless we understand we are no better than those we serve. There but for the Grace of God?

I am optimistic about the end of abortion and our current culture of death. I have seen people rethinking their past stand on abortion, reversing vasectomies, repentance, etc.

Maryland

The following information about the 1st Way (formerly Birthright) center in Maryland was contributed by Vicki Thornton, a 20 year volunteer, formerly for Birthright volunteer and currently for 1st Way. I have summarized and edited her story as appropriate, keeping as close to her own words as possible. Many of the same themes are present in her account including a personal calling to the work, community support and meeting women where they are with the acceptance of Christ.

The office was founded in 1974 response to a community effort to provide services for young women facing unplanned pregnancies. Since founder, Susan Bell, had been involved in a program outreach in another area, she felt called to begin a Birthright ministry locally. In addition, concerned community leaders representing various agencies and religious leaders offered to assist in her efforts.

The primary political challenge in Maryland was the climate of free choice for young women. It was considered important when counseling not to attract attention to the political debate over abortion rights. In fact, if one were involved in Right to Life publicity photos, that individual was discouraged from becoming a Birthright volunteer because it was assumed the individual could not offer objective views to the client.

The office was donated by a pro-life Baptist church group. This was their way of helping protect the lives of pre-born children. The office was overcrowded and filled with donated bags and boxes of maternity clothes and baby items. Funds were raised to keep the office going via church outreach requests. At one time, a newsletter listed prayer request items and these requests were often filled promptly once church boards became aware of those needs. Folks found out about the Center via word of mouth and some ads in the paper and phone book. Later, we tried to promote 1st Way in a college newspaper but our ad was rejected by the liberal editors.

The true mission of 1st Way is to offer an environment that is loving and without judgment. The Maryland center also offers an educational component to help young ladies identify their personal strengths and needs via a series of modules. All of these efforts are purely on a request basis; none of these programs are forced on the client.

Many of the volunteers are motivated by the Christian principle of reaching out to the most innocent of us all, the pre-born child. This outreach can be confirmed by ensuring that the Mom and other family members are able to continue with a crisis or unwanted pregnancy through outside assistance. This assistance is available based on the individual need of the client. Some volunteers are motivated by a past experience with her own unplanned pregnancy or abortion. Everyone called to this ministry is dedicated and appreciated. Personal rewards come from the realization of saving a baby's life and ministering to a mom and family in crisis.

The secret of touching the hearts of pregnant women in crisis is to act, as Jesus would have us act. Simply put, "What would Jesus do if he were a volunteer at 1st Way"? He would not judge, reprimand, punish or require penance. Jesus would extend His hand in love to mom and baby through the 9-month pregnancy and ensure that appropriate safeguards were there after the baby's birth.

Pro-lifers need to realize that they must walk the walk in addition to talking the talk. If we encourage alternatives to abortion, then we need to be there to ensure that such alternatives are available. Surely, the abortionists are available. Therefore, our presence is mandatory. 1st Way offered the umbrella philosophy that our Center was seeking so it was a perfect fit for our community.

I received my personal passion of love for the unborn at age 13. At that age, I learned that my 17-year old mom and her family had tried to "do away" with me. This was 63 years ago and there were no ultra sounds machines to reveal that I was alive and kicking. They only knew that my mom was too young to have a child. Obviously, and thankfully, their efforts failed. But my experience gave me an insight and heart for the pre-born child. It is hard to know how many babies have received the gift of life from our efforts. Even if it is only one, our efforts are worth all of the time and energy devoted to this cause. The Center nearly closed 4 years ago. Prayer and God's grace kept it open.

I remain very optimistic about the future of our Center because it is committed to the work of God. He has called a very dedicated Center Director, Virginia Cliff, to serve the clients and her heart and efforts have brought new life and enthusiasm to the Center. While the act of abortion by desperate and uninformed women may always occur, technology offers promise through the advancement of fetal development awareness. Technology will also help educate men and women about pro-life alternatives to abortion and provide information on crisis pregnancy centers. We have much work to do but we must be there to "stand in the gap" for babies and parents in need.

Arizona

The story of the clinic in Phoenix, Arizona was contributed by Maria Campion and echoes the stories of Eugene, Kansas, and others in the power of volunteers to get an office running.

Maria Campion and some women friends in Scottsdale and Tempe, realizing their legislators were pushing to create laws that would allow abortion in 1971-1972 attended their State Senate Hearings. They bravely stood before this body giving short speeches in defense of life, the principles of our country and their faith.

In addition, their group wrote letters and spoke to congressmen. But, when the idea of giving practical service to girls and women was presented to the Scottsdale group by a Birthright volunteer of Tucson, Maria Campion's group was energized. "We valued those who could lobby, debate and educate about the pro-life movement but some of us were drawn to the personal involvement with the girls who were suffering agonizing decisions about abortion," said Maria.

And so they began, assigning specific tasks to small groups. Some collected baby and maternity clothes, some researched where they could provide the service they wanted to do, some struggled with the writing of the constitution and by-laws. Activities were growing on kitchen tables, home desks, and picnic tables. Whenever there were a few minutes, they were formulating specific plans. They established and staffed a 24-hour hotline before they even had an office. They hired an answering service that put the call through to their homes and sometimes had to retreat to the shower stall in the bathroom to have the quiet and privacy to talk with a young woman contemplating abortion.

They were busy well before the Supreme Court decision of 1973. Planned Parenthood was sending girls from Arizona to California to have their abortions at that time. One of their first BR cases was a young woman who came back with serious complications. She called at 10:00 p.m., bleeding in a phone booth, and one of the doctor members saw her that very night because it was after hours at Planned Parenthood and their phone was not being answered. "That situation gave great inspiration to our group," Maria said.

"In the early years we wandered from place to place. First, upstairs in the Western Savings Building in Tempe, then at the old Kino Institute Building on Northern Avenue, then in a little duplex adjacent to the Diocesan Center, then to our house on West Thomas Road, then to the building at Phoenix College that had housed the Newman Center. Always the orphans, always knowing that our lease could run out at any time."

In spite of the wandering, their numbers grew and they attended conferences around the country and became more sophisticated in their practices. "We were privileged to create an environment of love in which mothers could hear the truth and choose life for their babies. One of the great blessings of those days was the rich encounter with people who shared our values and with whom deep and lasting friendships were established. It is with great joy that I read the First Way Newsletter. [I] see the sophistication of how things run now and notice that [the] same deep threads of faith and love are what inspire today's work as they inspired us so many years ago. God bless each one of you for the sacrifices you make for the lives of clients and their babies. And God bless each of your family members who generously share you with the suffering world."

Utah

I knew Sally Carr personally through conferences and admired her greatly. I have written the following about the Salt Lake City center based on my own knowledge and connection with Sally, who has now passed on. Sally's story is evidence of how much the director can impact the whole center with her inspiration. She is also a walking example of the nurturing love that Birthright centers hope to offer their clients.

Sally Carr is a wife and nurse and was director of the Salt Lake City Birthright for many years. Sally, by her own description was a giant of a woman who wore size 10 shoes, weighed nearly 200 pounds, had snow white hair and was a native New Yorker. But she was a gentle giant who possessed that calming presence and peace in every word. She was given to sighing deeply before answering a question put to her. There followed an astute assessment and often a new look at the situation. She was the one who admonished us to listen. "Ask questions because [you] wish to learn," she would say. This was her advice for the initial meeting with a woman. "We want to be available. We want to draw her out by writing down her important problems and gradually work with her to find solutions. It should be our goal to help the woman connect with her baby in the womb and find her own capabilities to confront her problems with our friendship as a support." Sally lived her words of advice. She made it her business to know all about welfare aid in her city and nationwide, for that matter.

The Clinton White house and their anti-life objectives were no mystery to her. "Hill and Billary" was her descriptive characterization. She was up on legislation and how the "system" works, on how to approach the doctors to enlist their help in caring for our women. My first recollection of Sally was her invitation to come to Salt Lake City to attend a board meeting. She wanted help to assess the qualities of the board and add the vision of BR to the floundering and questioning members. Sally wanted reinforcement of the charter goals. As Regional Consultant, I was able to help her in that need.

Sally Carr, now with God, summed up the goal of her Salt Lake City Center: "We are 100% service. We are dealing day by day with women who are pregnant or think they might be and are worried about that. We do the work that needs to be done, that's all." Speaking of office staff she said, "There are all kinds of people here but all volunteers. Nobody is practicing a profession. This is a grassroots, people-to-people kind of operation. We are practical: Do you have food? A safe place to live? Clothing for your baby? Women will continue to be pregnant without being sure they want to be. They will need to talk it out with somebody who will help them find what they need so they can make it. This is a human problem. We are outside of the political debate. But we are inside the problem."

Montana

Nancy Morton contributed this information about the center in Missoula. Her story illustrates that internal struggles with volunteers and with the charter were, sadly, widespread. Yet it also shows how the women called to this work are just ordinary people, following their hearts and a personal calling, with amazing results.

Nancy Morton is the founder of the Birthright center in Missoula, Montana. While caring for her 3-month old infant, Nancy passed the time one afternoon in 1976 by watching the Phil Donohue show on her TV. Amazingly, Phil was interviewing a guest from the National Right to Life office. He was telling about a group that offered alternatives to abortion. Nancy was instantly impressed and called her local parish priest to ask about information on this group. A National Right to Life convention just happened to be coming to town that very weekend. Nancy attended and spoke to the representative from the alternatives group. Also in attendance was a college student who shared interest in getting an office in Missoula and both were given rough copies of a manuscript of the founder's life and struggles, the story of Birthright. By the time Nancy finished the copy, her collaborator had moved on but she believed in the project of women helping others in crisis so she proceeded to canvass local churches for support. Almost as a last resort she attended a meeting of a small church. The little group of twelve was so enthusiastic that that very evening after he talk and plea, $1,200.00 was given to her to start. A small office was found and people like the Knights of Columbus donated furniture: a couch, desk and telephone. Some friends joined together to form a staff and the office opened in 1977 for two mornings a week.

Her first client was a woman grieving over the relinquishment of her child. No counseling had been given (these were still the days of closed adoption) and she confided to Nancy that she wondered every night if "my baby is cold." Nancy offered her positive encouragement with the present pregnancy. At the birth the mother and Nancy shared great joy.

During her 13-year tenure as director Nancy faced difficulties with a woman in her office that wished to change the focus of Birthright to one that would include and stress proselytizing. A confrontation led to both women leaving the center. Fortunately, board members were determined to carry on and they, and a new director, guided the office. They continued to find new directors and, by 2003, an Executive Director was found who also agreed to help with the use of an ultrasound that had been a gift of Focus on the Family. Their center is thriving today and financial worries are not part of their future.

Illinois

The contribution from Connie Freund in McHenry Illinois reveals the same pattern of grassroots beginnings. The struggle to find a long term location and the gathering of volunteers who must balance their own families with their work are common themes to so many Birthright stories.

The founder of Birthright in McHenry was a woman by the name of Barbara Svodboda, who moved from South Dakota where she had also started a Birthright. She was followed by Tina Gorski and then by me, the current director, Connie Freund. Together with the pastor of St. Mary's Church, she invited interested parishioners to a meeting on starting a pregnancy care center. At that time the pastor did not want it known that he supported the center even though he firmly believed as a Catholic priest that abortion was wrong.

As a mother of six children, I could not believe Roe V. Wade was passed and a mother could kill her unborn child. I felt so strongly about it that I went to that first meeting held at St. Mary's to get information on what I could do. From there, Birthright began and in December 1978 it was incorporated in Illinois. Shortly after the center opened in Barb Svoboda's living room, we moved to a one room rent free office space above a real estate company. From there we moved to professional offices, a house, another office, a house, and then to the present location. It began with six volunteers from St. Mary's Church who volunteered a few hours each week. I was there one evening every other week by myself. We had a desk, two chairs, a file cabinet and a telephone. Now when one walks into our center they are surprised and comforted by the interior. The knotty pine walls, a large wooden staircase leading to the "Mommy's Treasures" gift shop, and the comfortable couches all radiate warmth. This is the welcoming characteristic we have sought to express from the lighting to the rugs on the floor.

Funds were raised though Mother's Day flower sales - red roses available for a donation of $1 - at six area Catholic churches. Donations of maternity clothing, baby furniture, and infant clothing were received after we moved to the next rented location.

In the April 1980 newsletter, *The Delivery*, Birthright was described as:

...the local chapter of an international organization offering free emergency service to pregnant women. Based on the notion that every pregnant woman has the right to give birth and every child has the right to be born. Birthright offers positive alternatives to abortion and help to women of all ages, married or single, who chose to continue pregnancy. Birthright in a volunteer, non-sectarian, non-profit, organization operating a crisis center where any concerned person can find help as available as the nearest telephone. It is manned by volunteers, and backed by counselors and social service agencies.

Birthright does not counsel for abortions or distribute birth control information of any kind at any time. We do not compete with existing health and social service programs, but make use of all existing programs under federal, state, and private sponsorship which are designed to assist the expectant mother.

Birthright volunteers are dedicated to bringing together the distressed woman and the people who are waiting to help her. They will inform them of the services available in the community in the hope that the woman faced with and unexpected pregnancy, and under the pressures of society to obtain an abortion quickly, will seek alternatives before making a decision - to be fair to herself and her unborn child.

There is never a charge for Birthright services for the pregnant woman or her family. Birthright tries to meet the needs of individuals, offering a friendly ear and a helping hand to a woman in need, while referring pregnancy related problems to the proper agencies. All calls are confidential.

Birthright is funded by contributions from individuals and organizations as well as the hours of donated services of the Birthright volunteers who work without pay.

People important to me were fellow Birthright volunteers who gave so much of their time. For example Alice, a wife and mother of ten children, who believed strongly in helping the distressed pregnant women through one-to-one contact as a way to face the abortion issue head on. Also Barbara, who was willing to start a second pregnancy center right after moving into a new area and not knowing anyone. She demonstrated much courage and love. And of course, God, my husband, and my six children all supported me. Only through my faith in God and belief that all life is sacred, from the womb to the tomb, have I been able to continue to help women in need of support during their pregnancies.

Yes, There was one time I felt I should stop and let someone else take over. It was when we lost our lease at a location where we had spent several years. It was our fourth center since 1978 and we had to find a new place in the same area so we could keep our same telephone number since 1978. I almost gave up but prayed for guidance. Well, a place was found and kept us open for two years before our board member found a better location in a home in Johnsburg in 2000. Last year we had to move again across the street to a very comfortable center for our clients and volunteers. So even though we have moved several times over the last 29 years, I am still here and very happy to be there for the moms and their babies.

Over the past 29 years there have been hundreds of volunteers and several have stayed over 18 years. I am very thankful for each and every one that spent whatever time they could. Almost all had gifts to share with out moms. Only a few did not and they did not last. If concerns came up regarding difficult situations, I always tried to have the volunteer understand our mission: "To provide loving assistance, emotional, and financial support for women and girls who find themselves in a crisis pregnancy."

Traveling to conventions was a highlight I looked forward to and I attended as many as I could including Toronto, Ottawa, Montreal, Notre Dame, Cherry Hill, Philadelphia, Denver, Chicago, Columbus, Myrtle Beach, Reno, Los Angeles, Albuquerque, and Oklahoma. As director, the center recently paid for my expenses and in the past the center has paid for volunteer's registration when funds were available. To encourage attendance to the conferences, we continue to offer to pay for the registration fees. Other than conference expenses, we have never had paid staff.

The Birthright charter was followed because we believed in it. When the problems and eventual split occurred after Louise Summerfield's failing health and the change in command, Denise and the USA board were not treated fairly. Instead, Canada took their grievances to court and Denise lost not only the Birthright USA name, but also her recognition as the first USA leader to reach out to women and offer life and the 1st Way for their unborn babies.

It was difficult to change the name from Birthright to 1st Way in 1994 because people thought we were no longer available. Because of our belief in Denise and the life saving ministry she directed, we felt the need to be an affiliate of National Life Center, to stand up for her support of the unborn in the United States. Even though other Birthright centers did not become affiliates, they continued to do the same work in their centers and supported Denise as well.

Word of mouth, Churches, newspaper articles, flower sales and other fundraisers helped to spread the word of our services in the community. The older women who called were easier to talk to as they listened better and were more likely to reason before decision making. The younger girls required faster talk to reach them because they were prone to panic quickly and are heavily influenced by peer pressure.

Our office has grown considerably: trained volunteers, clerical, layette & maternity clothing, "Mommy's Treasures" gift shop, Earn while you learn prenatal classes in both English and Spanish, and fundraising - Baby Bottle Boomerang, flower sales, baby showers, plant sales, Heaven & Earth Club, donations for doctors expenses and many miscellaneous fundraisers held by individuals, churches and organizations.

Our mission is to console women who find themselves in an unplanned or planned pregnancy, with the support and help they need to give birth to their unborn child. I feel we are able to share services that are available in our community to help them financially and/or emotionally. Listening to each woman and showing concern for her needs is our focus each time the telephone rings or she comes into the center.

Volunteer counselor training is provided on a one-to-one with the director and committed volunteer who has been on staff for at least one year. The training period is normally six weeks, meeting once a week for two to three hours. A training manual is followed step by step during the six weekly sessions to help the volunteer meet the needs of the pregnant mom and learn office procedures. There are times when they start as a receptionist and get their feet wet , so to speak, then in depth training follows. Depending on the needs of our center, many volunteers are not trained to counsel but do office work, cleaning, sort clothing, prepare layette, maintain the gift shop, prepare the newsletter, and mailings to name a few of the jobs available.

Volunteer meetings are held four times a year, one being the Christmas party. Each meeting is held on a Saturday for three hours, including s light lunch, and includes a speaker from some of our community services to keep us up on support available in our area. Our office hours are normally 9am to 3 or 4 pm four days a week, half a day on Fridays, one evening every other week, and three hours on Saturdays. To fill these hours our volunteers are asked to spend three hours a week. It is through God and his Holy Spirit that our volunteers can do what they do. they work very well together and help each other in many ways in the office and in other areas.

In order to keep up our enthusiasm we also have fun together. Our 1st Way board is a big support to me. I can call upon them when needs arise and they are willing to help. I do feel at times that the board should take more control as they seem to let me direct them at time. Perhaps that can be a good thing though. I am still looking out for a new director to take my place. Some one who works with me and will continue helping this center grow as needed.

We choose to minister to every woman who comes in our door no matter where she has come from or what she has. Those who do not want to listen; we need to be a friend to them. There is a saying I learned in Cursillo: "Make a friend, be a friend, and bring that friend to Christ." We do not proselytize at 1st Way but this statement can be used to reach out. Make them your friend and then be their friend. We simply do this by listening to them and staying in touch with them even when it is difficult.

When someone asks me what 1st Way is, I have to stop and again realize that we need to do more to increase awareness in our area and across the country. Our office now answers the phone with 1st Way Life Center" to increase awareness of what we do. More reaching out with the 1st Way message needs to be done through advertising. The more the word gets out, the more others will want to be a part of 1st Way. I struggle with how to do this. Should we network with CareNet or Heartbeat international to get the word out? What are the other ways available? At the same time I want to stay the way we are because of what we do for our clients.

I believe women will always need some type of support during their pregnancies and I see us continuing even after the end of abortion.

We need to continue to fight for the end of abortion and the culture of death, to change our country back to a culture of life!

Connie began as a volunteer with several other women at St. Mary's in McHenry in 1978, at the grassroots of Birthright in McHenry and has remained with the crisis pregnancy center since that time. In the beginning, she raised 6 sons with her husband and didn't have much time to spend at Birthright. Slowly, over the years, her desire to continue kept her more active. In 2008 they are in the process of growing once again.

New Jersey

This very simple contribution from the center in New Jersey seems an appropriate close to this chapter. When asked why it is important to accept the pregnant woman without judgment, even those called "unreachable," West Collingwood, New Jersey, 1st Way Director, Cass Farrell said, "I think it is in the heart of the volunteer to keep close to God and ask for Grace. We are simply there for the girl/woman who comes to us. When I feel like leaving or am afraid I pray for perseverance, so I pray all of the time. In the meantime, I pray for the end of abortion and will do all I can for the babies."

Another Perspective, by Denise Cocciolone

The Birth of a New Idea

There has arisen within the pro-life movement a phenomenon called the Crisis Pregnancy Center (CPC). Over 3,000 of these centers are now operating in the USA and countries around the world. Many thousands of volunteers have taken up their posts to assist pregnant women who choose to give their children life. Political coverage of the abortion debate is widespread, yet these clinics have stood on the front lines defending the dignity of life with amazingly little public notice or media attention. It may seem like the only people who know about and use these service centers are the women distressed by an untimely pregnancy. These centers are staffed by ordinary people, supported by a few savvy donors who have caught the vision of how a grassroots endeavor could be used to halt the behemoth of abortion and provide a peaceful and dignified future to mothers and babies. Even so these centers have had a transformative effect on many lives if we will but read the statistics. Abortions are down.

The beauty of the person-to-person approach came about through the inspiration of the founder, Louise Summerhill, and has been carried forth by her USA counterpart, Denise Cocciolone. These two women forged a path to what is now known as the pro-life service movement. Because Louise has already written her book on the beginning of the Birthright movement in Canada, The Story of Birthright, it is worthwhile to give some thought to the second woman, her partner, Denise. Her story parallels the crisis pregnancy center movement itself and to share her story is to share the history of the volunteer staffed centers whose miraculous accomplishments have changed thousands of lives, yet have never basked in the glow of mainstream media attention.

Denise carried out Louise's idea by presenting the steps necessary for a pregnancy center to find a place on earth: A place which invites distressed women to enter. According to Denise, the tone/ impressions given during the initial contact sets the tone for how she's going to see her future and how she's going to see the child. The office, although sharing some characteristics of business offices with telephones, chairs, brochures, a desk and couches, is a unique place because it is to facilitate a friendly, non-threatening encounter. An encounter between a worried woman and an accomplished person who possesses a sincere desire to lighten the pregnant woman's burden by providing practical resources and the courage to help her mobilize her own resources, as well. If the pregnant woman wants, the volunteer will follow the pregnant woman every step of the way on her journey to motherhood, whether in the end she chose to parent or give her baby life through adoption. To keep a network of small offices nationwide up and running is a daunting task. It's definitive voluntary character depends on the good will of staff members. With absolutely no political backing, this grassroots movement placed itself squarely against the prevailing culture of death with its worship of abortion as the sacrament of freedom. With the insouciance of a crusader confident in the truth of her cause, Denise became a fearless leader for the culture of life in the United States. She was always ready to encourage and provide a practical, no nonsense approach to the daily problems of Birthright clinics around the country from her headquarters in New Jersey.

The makeup of an alternatives-to-abortion group such as Birthright, was for the most part homemakers, who while living the demands of family life, would add an additional challenge to their busy lives. To fight abortion and help pregnant women, these wives and mothers would have to rouse themselves and go to an office 3 hours weekly. While volunteers were distinctly independent thinkers they refused to accept the status quo of abortion, but they were not politically ambitious types. For most, new skills had to be acquired to fulfill their tasks. Methods of active listening, stages of fetal development, and abortion techniques were just a few of the areas they had to study. Sr. Paula Vandegaer furnished much of this training with media tapes instruction. Volunteers were be required to spend many precious hours in intense training, as they made the necessary sacrifices to keep to their posts in all life's trying circumstances. The very first pregnant woman Denise helped was a foreign exchange student deserted by her boyfriend.

Through hard work and intuition, Denise became a resource for other pro-life groups who wanted to start a national hotline. Always willing to lend a hand and give practical advice to smooth the way, Denise became a well known person in the pro-life movement early on.

From the beginning, in 1970, Denise used her considerable talents to organize and promote the Birthright concept with a single-minded enthusiasm. Her commitment to all of the unborn and their mothers took shape in high goals that she challenged volunteers to meet, volunteers whom she was ultimately in charge of as USA director. She knew these challenges would bring out the very best in the centers' staff. The center workers, in turn, responded with verve but at times in frustration. The continuous demands of service to an office day in and day out for years made for serious soul searching. Some people could not sustain the rigors. Offices faced heavy staff turnover.

In private life, Denise was equally searching for perfection in herself. She and her husband, Johnny, could have easily qualified for international competition in ballroom dancing. She and husband Johnny are parents of two adopted children. They took the duties and responsibilities of parenthood seriously and were grateful for the lives that were permitted to live to make their own family. Denise Cocciolone could best be described as one at the center of controversy. A natural redhead, she is also a true radical. As a teen she opted to remain in an unheated house while the rest of her family relocated to a house in another part of town because she wanted to finish high school with her own class. She converted to Catholicism independently because of the good example of some of her girlfriends. She married a man not to her mother's liking. Then, as a wife and mother, Denise involved herself in the greatest controversy of the century: abortion.

Denise became president of her local Right To Life group to help change peoples hearts on abortion. She had witnessed the tragic outcomes when two of her friends procured clandestine abortions in high school. She vowed to help other women by preventing the spread of abortion. She had confided in her pastor that she had read an article in her local Catholic newspaper about the idea of establishing alternatives to abortion and this had stirred her interest. Two of her fellow pro-lifers, Carmine Pecorelli, Executive Director of New Jersey's RTL and Joe McCullough, lawyer, urged Denise to go to a Minnesota conference to meet a lady with the big idea for helping pregnant women.

Denise did attend that conference and met Birthright founder Louise Summerhill. She says that the idea of ordinary people reaching out to help at the crucial moment of decision was fascinatingly appealing. It was a simple idea practical help that appealed to me. I could do this organize an office. It was within my reach, said Denise.

Louise invited Denise to the final drafting of the Birthright Charter in 1971 in Scarborough, Canada. Also in attendance were Bernadette Sanders of Kansas, Dr. Charles Hillabrand of Ohio, and Sr. Paula Vandegaer of California. Louise looked forward to collaboration with these people. Once at home in Ohio, Dr. Hillabrand moved to propose a person of his own choosing, a Holocaust survivor Lorie Maie, as president of alternatives to abortion, Louise felt a personal heartbreak. The doctor's plans were ultimately rejected, however, including his proposal of establishing headquarters for the new group in Columbus, Ohio. Louise moved quickly to put Denise in the position of Director of Birthright USA by December 1971, with herself as director in Canada. During that year centers opened in Oregon, Virginia and Kansas with the support of Louise in Toronto.

Denise put her hand to the task before her to organize, inform and disseminate the concept of Birthright in the United States. Louise kept busy inspiring her fellow countrymen to join the cause of protecting unborn babies by offering practical help. It was an exhilarating time for both women. Denise tells the story of spending and entire night writing response letters to interested groups. By 5 a.m. she was caught up only to realize that in 5 more hours a flood of mail would be pouring into her office for responses.

Denise possessed an intuitive outlook on how and where help was needed as well as how to apply this knowledge in the most succinct, yet gentle and respectful manner. She tried to conveyed her approach to the various centers staffs with in-person meetings for the staff. Flying all over the United States she spread her upbeat message: "You can be of help because you know what abortion does and you have the means through practical friendship to guide the pregnant woman before you," said Denise.

Early in organizing the alternatives-to-abortion movement, representatives of the Catholic Bishops wanted to make Birthright a part of Catholic Charities with a Board of Directors and a more professional image. Both Louise and Denise agreed that the job of offering help was a job that housewives, mothers and grandmothers were fitted for because they could spend the extra hours that it would take to help women in distress outside of regular office times. As Denise says, crises usually do not occur during business hours and Birthright people could be free from constraints time-wise. They would also do things that professionals were not able or willing to do: clean an apartment, transport someone to the doctor, give out clothing, and talk at odd hours.

Other challenges to the abortion alternative approach appeared in the form of good and holy projects like Natural Family Planning (NFP). While she agreed that NFP was admirable for married couples, Denise recognized that Birthright clients were, for the most part, not involved in the stable marital relationship that this method required. The centers remained focused on the individual woman who is already pregnant, leaving other areas of education to other groups. One of the most persistent obstacles to the simple and streamlined approach of Birthright was the desire on the part of some states for a statewide board to oversee the small, local Birthright centers. Again, Denise helped Louise to see that state structures would only add a burden to the directors who would look upon the boards as another intermediate in their quest for answers and help from their ultimate source: Birthright in Canada.

Difficulties plagued Denise's life on her own turf. Her office in New Jersey was forced to move three times in the course of five years before finally settling into the present place in 1976. Money was a problem. Mortgage debts and moving costs had to be paid by scarce dollars garnered from friends. As a grass roots organization, Birthright paid no salaries to staff but depended solely on the love and commitment of people awake and aware of the tragedy that was unfolding before their very eyes. Husbands of the women volunteers even chipped in by moving furniture, painting, and donating funds.

The Structure of the Center System

Louise and Denise wanted to make the organization of Birthright as friendly as possible to housewives coming out of their kitchens. These women had to feel ownership in their centers. A family feeling developed very soon in Birthright. The all-volunteer staff depended much on each of their directors and the directors especially had to deal with feeling of being torn between responsibilities at home versus the office. That's where regional and national meetings were so helpful. At these meetings the leaders could freely discuss their burdens and receive consolation and fellowship. The idea of a Regional Consultant with responsibilities to her designated states was the brain child of Carmine Pecorelli, Executive Director of Right To Life in New Jersey. With this person, a personal contact with particular regional needs was provided.

Denise attended many Regional State meetings. She could sympathize with the feelings of stress of the staff. She summarized her own feelings when she described an incident with her oldest child, Vince, who was scheduled to make his first confession. That same night people in Princeton, NJ, expected to hear details of this brand new organization called Birthright and how they could open an office in their community. Denise says she cried all the way to Princeton from her home in Woodbury although she knew her sister-in-law and mother-in-law would be in attendance for her son. How many times such wrenching decisions were made by Louise, Denise and the vast numbers of Birthright people who had made their vows to help end the scourge of abortion in their life time! On one occasion Denise was being interviewed by a reporter and was asked, Why do you do this? Before she could answer, her little toddler daughter, Jennifer, began to sing in her child's voice a nursery song, ABCDEFG. Delighted, Denise pointed to Jen and said, That's why I do this, so others can live and sing and have a good life.

Some relief from the silent rigors of the abortion wars came from the White House itself. When Ronald Reagan became President, Louise and Denise received invitations to speak about Birthright. As Louise's representative, Denise testified before Congress during Jeremiah Denton's tenure in 1982. Her final meeting was in 1988 when several Birthright directors and other pro-life representatives were invited to the Oval Office for a personal meeting with the President. There never was another time for such public acceptance of an organization like Birthright. The media blackout for abortion alternatives had already begun, so here, at least, was some recognition of the work accomplished.

The international Birthright conventions held every June, alternately in Canada or the US, were also wonderful events. The financial difficulties of attending these sites made the gathering all the more fruitful. Some women traveled long hours by bus. There were hundreds of Birthright people from all parts of the US and Canada at these meetings that included inspiring and informative pro-life speakers from every part of the Right To Life movement. There were specialists in counseling, medicine, fundraising and advertising. These were the uplifts that were needed in the daily struggle and it was Denise and her staffs that coordinated and developed these programs every year for 20 years.

The Growth of the Life Movement

From 1971 to 1980 we saw many other groups with pro-life agendas blossom and grow. There was the Right To Life organization of the late 1960s, the Right to Life Committee formed in May of 1973, and political action groups at all state levels. The American Life League was founded by Judie Brown in 1984 and the March for Life was formed by Nellie Gray in 1974 and continues to gather huge crowds in Washington DC even today.

When asked her opinion on so many groups, Denise characteristically affirmed that pro-life people are strong willed and diverse. There are thousands of people doing various things in the pro-life movement. Does that mean that the movement is hurt or fragmented? No! Everyone has a certain personality makeup. Perhaps our work in the crisis pregnancy centers is too quiet for some. There is need for everyone's talents. The movement has even attracted kooks but they are not truly pro-life.

With Louise's permission Denise set up a 24/7 hotline to cover all the United States. This was the first of its kind anywhere in the world. The national hotline was staffed by a live person who could direct women to their nearest pro-life pregnancy center while giving as much time as needed. It required a great deal of money to set up and maintain telephone lines adequate to the task. In addition, it required paid employees to staff the phones and there was a tremendous need for more income to support this endeavor. Needing more money meant bringing fundraising to an entirely new level.

Changes in Canadian laws created chaos. For example, in 1990 the Canadian Government passed a law concerning non-profit organizations that caused Louise to notify all centers to stop talking about abortion to the client unless the client herself brought up the topic. This policy change was very troublesome to the centers in the United States. Birthright USA was becoming known by more and more clients and supporters. Donors saw Birthright as a good way to quell abortions in this country. One great success was when Birthright USA was given enough money to purchase ads in the Readers Digest. They read: 10 good reasons why she cant have this baby. Birthright took care of all of them.

In 1990 a falling out had occurred between Louise and Denise and Louise conferred the title of Co-Director of Birthright USA upon another consultant, Terry Weaver of Georgia and in August of 1991 Louise died. These sudden events left Denise uncertain of her own position in Birthright USA, but to the world, the service movements successes continued. In 1992 Denise and I were invited by the Right To Life committee to go to the newly opened countries of Lithuania and Russia to give talks on how to start a Birthright center. It was the ultimate irony for Denise to play her role as Birthright director overseas and then return to the United States to face the decidedly perplexing question of who was in charge of Birthright USA. After Louise's death, her daughters favored Terry Weaver for Director in the United States. Denise was under the mistaken impression that she could continue to share the BR trademark name because of her long standing with the organization.

For two years there were meetings, negotiations and, unfortunately, a court battle. In the end, Denise lost the right to use the Birthright name. Denise, once so confident, felt the ground shake beneath her.

She renamed her center the National Life Center, and groups affiliated with her were called 1st Way. While the work was the same, it had to be done in a vastly different set of circumstances with a change in name and affiliation. It was a heartbreaking testament to the fallible humanity of even those who dedicate their lives to serving others.

Denise has remained steadfast at her post in New Jersey, tenaciously keeping to the original concept of Birthrights alternatives to abortion. The anguish has taken its toll. While there is still a national convention and hotline, there are centers with different names, fewer volunteers and donors and, consequently, fewer reasons to get together. Denise has held on to the support of Congressman Chris Smith and Fr. Frank Pavone and her center directors still call upon her for advice and counsel.

Modern Times and Challenges for Crisis Pregnancy Centers

In recent years 1st Way centers have faced many challenges. Client loads are down because of the name change. There are reliable home tests and there has been a proliferation of high school based health clinics where teens are provided birth control pills. Crisis pregnancy centers are widely accepted and used by county health departments to share the load of pregnancy testing. However, the media has steadfastly ignored their presence in communities. Even the Internet has worked against the old face to face contact of volunteers with pregnant women. Now, a woman can access an abortionist from the privacy of her home computer, buy over the counter Plan B or have a prescription for RU486.

On the other hand, ultrasounds have helped draw interested and curious pregnant women to make appointments with a volunteer counselor. In some states crisis pregnancy centers are busier than ever. The Wichita Kansas office, Birthline, does over 1,000 tests per year. With its greater financial support, CareNet centers are practically taking over the service movement. In addition, the original group started by Dr. Hillabrand in 1971 has renamed and reformed itself into the large and growing organization called Heartbeat International with centers in many parts of the world. These centers are well staffed, mostly by paid professional social workers rather than volunteers.

These two groups, CareNet and Heartbeat now represent the bulk of the centers performing pregnancy care. Both have tweaked the original concept of alternatives to abortion staffed by ordinary women. Their additional burden of an evangelical agenda sometimes seems to overshadow the original simple desire to help women in crisis. This cannot help but remind one of the Catholic nuns at the turn of the century who created and staffed hospitals and orphanages. These dedicated women were supplanted by professional social workers in the 1930s and 1940s. The nuns were dismissed as incompetent because they did not carry educational degrees. Though the trend away from concerned individuals toward trained professionals is somewhat disconcerting, it is heartening to see that the movement continues to grow, gently calling our culture back to the precious gift of life.

Denise has kept abreast of the continuous outpouring from feminist literary stars like Germaine Greer and Gloria Steinem who, aided and abetted by Planned Parenthood's subsidized Kaye Wattleton's propaganda, have been part of the grim anti-life landscape. Denise has been aware that powerful political groups like NOW and NARAL have emerged to further challenge and attack CPCs but she always points to talented pro-life feminists (e.g., Daphne deJong, Rosemary Bottcher, Denise Handler, Mary Mehan) who have written their essays and testimonials and received some media attention for their stand against abortion. Slowly there is emerging a consensus that abortion does hurt women.

Many pro-life supporters have written books full of suggestions as to how pregnancy centers could change and do more to encourage pregnant women clients to place their babies for adoption, to get married to the father of their babies, or to stop abortion-minded women from going ahead with their firm plans. Denise would balance these with her steadfast understanding of our goals in the face of human weakness. The mothers life is a sacred as the baby's.

Denise did not succumb to any reliance on outside expertise. The well intentioned advice has usually lacked the intimate knowledge of the very human situations that center staff face. Concern over these suggestions has been offset by Denise's common sense assessment and encouragement. Unrealistic demands, Denise would call these attempts at improvements. Better to have faith in divine providence and leave our efforts at God's feet, she would reiterate.

A Woman to Remember: Sr. Paula Vandegaer

In 1968 Sister Paula, a professed Sister of Social Service in Los Angeles California, was helping a client who had recently placed her baby for adoption. The young lady was trying to decide whether artificial contraception would be a new part of her life. At that moment Sister received a clear vision of an incredible battle between the good of life vs. the terribly destructive force of this birth control pill. In one flash Sister's prescient sense was that the moral standards of society would be irrevocably damaged and degraded. Upon this awesome insight Sister knew that she would give all her own strength to help women and so many others to understand that their Godly identities as persons of worth and dignity must be guarded from this evil.

This insight became a hallmark of her long and fruitful career in pro-life work. In 1967 Colorado, North Carolina and California, Sisters home state, liberalized abortion laws. As the saying goes, politics is the art of the compromise. Governor Reagan of California, although torn by his deep regard for life, was forced by legislature head Jess Unruh to sign a bill allowing abortion in order to get his budget through the House. This was a decision he said he regretted always. With this capitulation on the State of California's part, Sister knew that she had to enter the battle against abortion. As a Sister of Social Service, she knew where her talents lay reaching out to distressed human beings, especially those considering abortion through counseling.

She called together five of her social work colleagues. Her vision was to put together a guide to help the many people who were eager to help pregnant women who would be tempted because of the relaxed restrictions on abortion to opt for the procedure.

Every two weeks for three months her friends and colleagues met to create a training manual that would be available to hundreds of lay people engaged in helping pregnant women. What would be the necessary elements of this manual? Her group came up with basic tools that were clear and yet fitted to the outreach of non-professionals.

In addition, Sister trained herself, trained and guided a group in Whittier, California, in the materials from the professional study groups training material. This was indeed an unprecedented accomplishment that non-professionals would undertake with her help.

In a few months many pro-life groups had heard about this manual. It was much in demand. Many ordinary citizens were determined to push back against the surging waves of abortion. Anyone who was awake and alive to the dangerous legal precedents began to band together to do something practical to help the distressed pregnant women.

By 1971 the RTL League of Southern California became aware that the entire Catholic Bishops Council under Msgr. McHugh was promoting and underwriting the first National Convention of Pregnancy Counseling Services in Washington, DC. Their network of Diocesan Family Life Office's prominent people made life issues the entire program. There were also unknown but eager and competent attendees like Louise Summerhill, Dr. Hillabrand, Lorie Maier, Denise Cocciolone, Bernadette Sanders and, of course, Sister Paula, with her professional credentials as counselor. There were over 60 groups represented at that historic meeting. The idea of creating and staffing a crisis pregnancy center in all parts of the country and Canada was deemed to be a worthwhile endeavor.

Louise came prepared with a very specific plan of how to establish and organize such a group. She invited interested people to a meeting with her staff to be held in Scarborough, Ontario a few months hence. Some of the participants, including Sr. Paula, took exception to some of Louise's priorities and operational procedures although both agreed on the pro-life theme of the centers. There were two different visions but always the goal of saving an unborn baby's life, said Sr. Paula.

Sister preferred a more open system where centers would always offer alternatives to abortion but would be free to organize themselves according to the operational procedures they though best suited to their groups. Back in the USA, Dr. Hillabrand, Lorie and Sister formed their own group known as Alternatives to Abortion International (AAI) with Lorie as Executive Director in Toledo, Ohio.

Alternatives to Abortion International

This grassroots movement of CPCs was gaining more and more adherents. Sr. estimates that two new centers opened every week! This was a phenomenal growth pattern that necessitated networking to keep and nurture unity. Sister accomplished this essential task again with the creation of a National Directory.

Her training manual to help centers to establish themselves on a professional foundation became an even more sought after commodity because the new centers knew they had to win the respect of medical communities in which they lived. By 1975 the work of Sister's organization headed by Lorie Maier was becoming an overwhelming task for one person. Lorie asked Sister, who was Secretary for the AAI Board, to come to Toledo to help out. Sister, of course, was unwilling to leave her own religious community but she told Lorie she could help her from Los Angeles. In what specific way? Under the power of inspiration, Sister decided that a well-produced magazine would be the answer to keep all the centers informed and inspired. Included in the journal were articles on timely and educational topics of a wide variety.

Heartbeat magazine, the pioneer publication of the pro-life movement was born! Later, its name changed to *Living World* but always, it provided vital information and inspiration to pro-lifers. In addition to all this magazine work on Sister's part, she decided to use another media stream, the videotape. In the 1980s Sister produced training tapes on every important topic for centers: confidentiality, basic attitudes of the counselor, etc.

She initiated a series of articles on the newly identified post abortion syndrome, found in research papers and reported in newspaper articles. This medical news showed that since Japanese citizens had experienced abortions since post WWII, there was a growing acknowledgment from psychologists and social scientists that causes of women's depression, anxiety and even ill health in general could be linked to Japans policy of abortion on demand. Post Abortion Stress (PAS) was likened to the illness of soldiers who returned from war with a whole panoply of symptoms related to the stress of combat experience.

By 1983 Lorie Maier retired and after a series of other Directors, Peggy Hartsborn was tapped as Executive Director in 1988. From that point the organization became known as Heartbeat International. It is a great organization with numerous centers.

Sister Paula decided to form her own group in 1985 known as International Life Service. Ever the innovator, her yearly meetings were called advanced training institutes because they focused on one subject to increase attendees skills. These institutes would study in depth one specific topic of interest essential to CPCs rather than many topics.

Yet another gift to the pro-life movement is Sister's creation of a live in community in the heart of Los Angeles where pro-life people take on the role of student interns for one or two years. They are engaged in the study of pro-life issues and enjoy hands on work in her center. Her goal for this Learning Center is to develop consistent, accomplished pro-life leaders to be the providers of alternatives to abortion to the ends of the earth so babies can be saved from abortion.

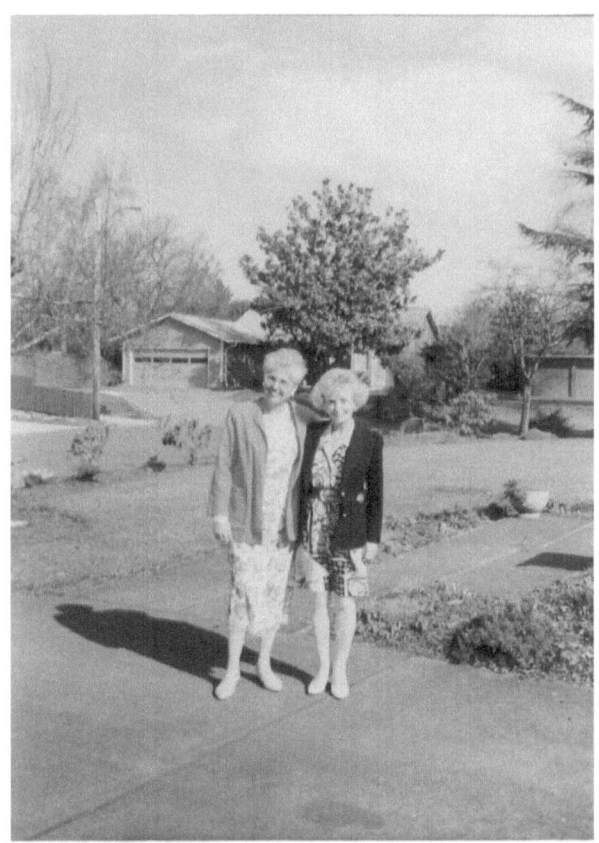

Denise Cocciolone
Pres.National Life Center
20th Anniversary Birthright, Eugene

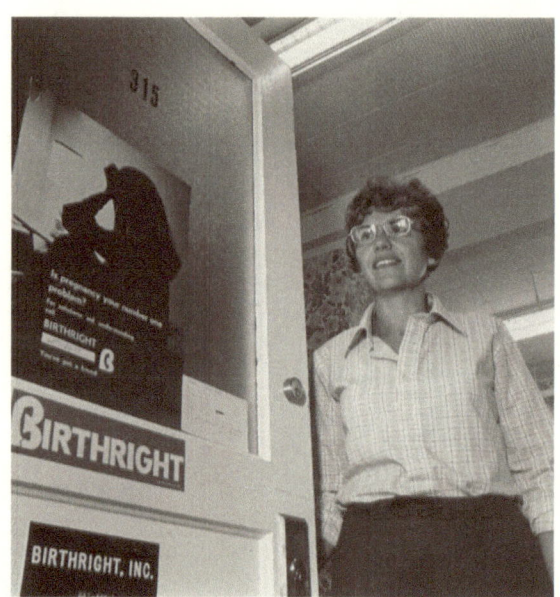

First Office

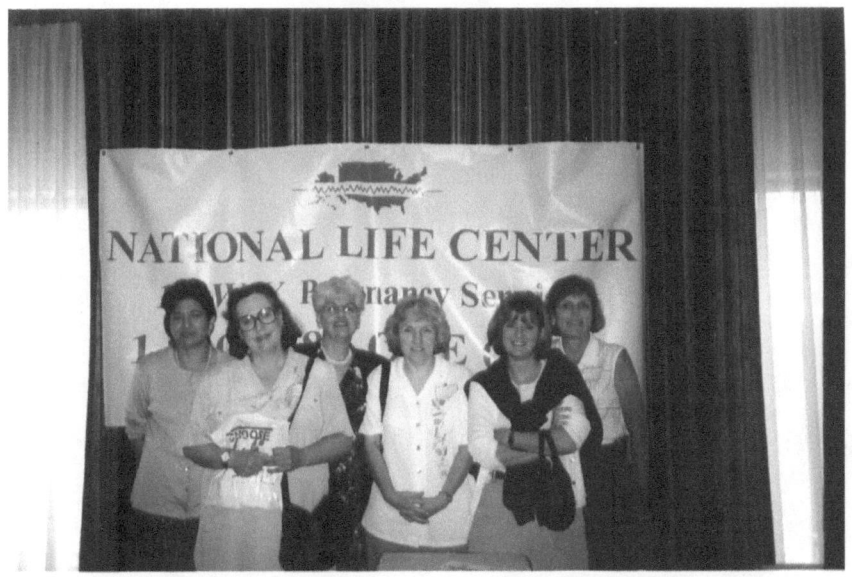

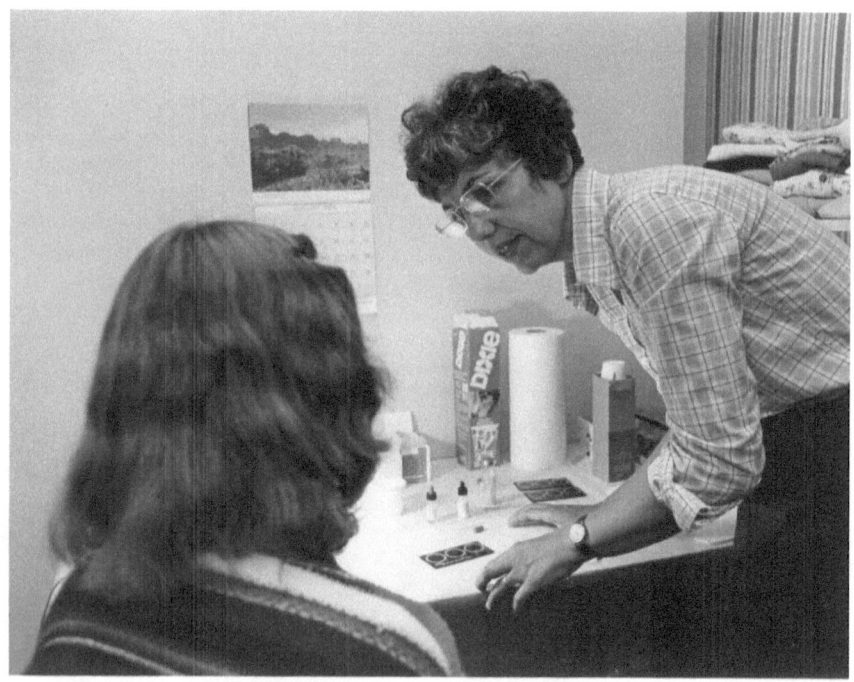

Old Pregnancy Tests 1976

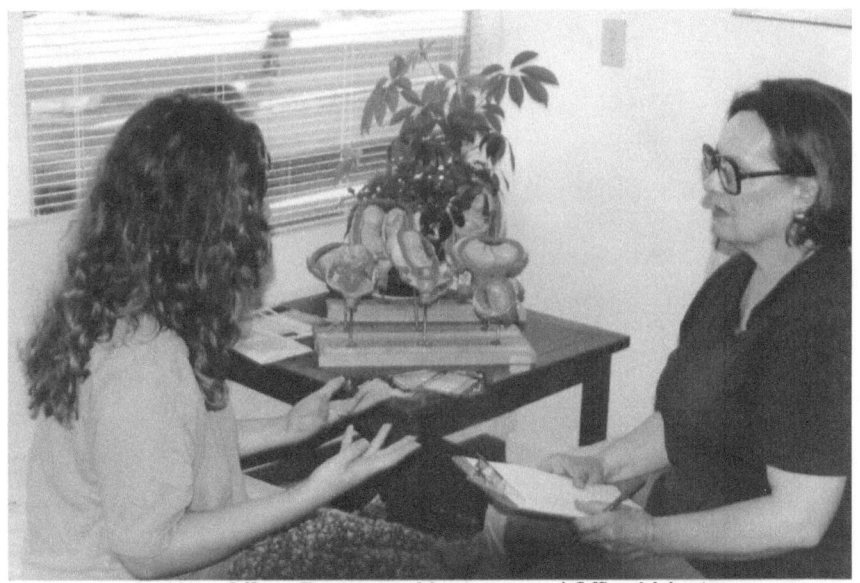

1st Way Office: Rosemary Montgomery / Office Volunteer

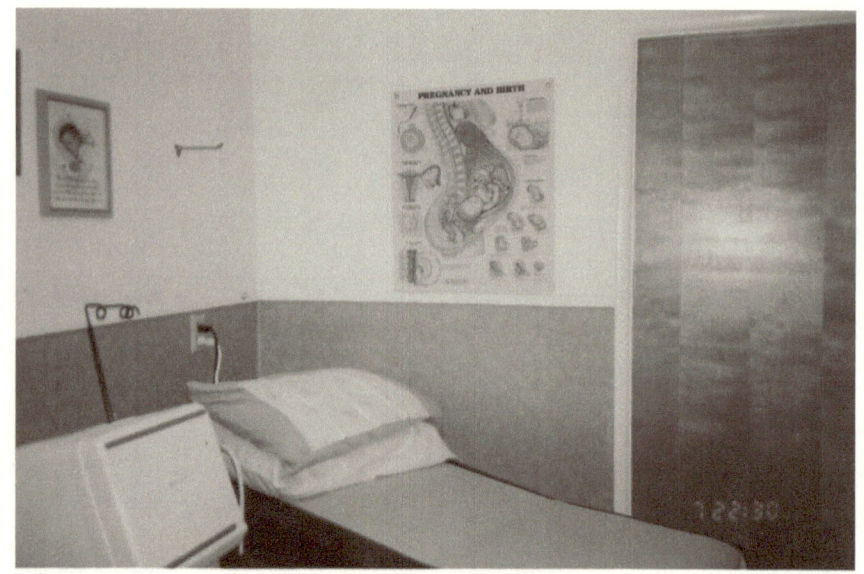

Ultra Sound Room

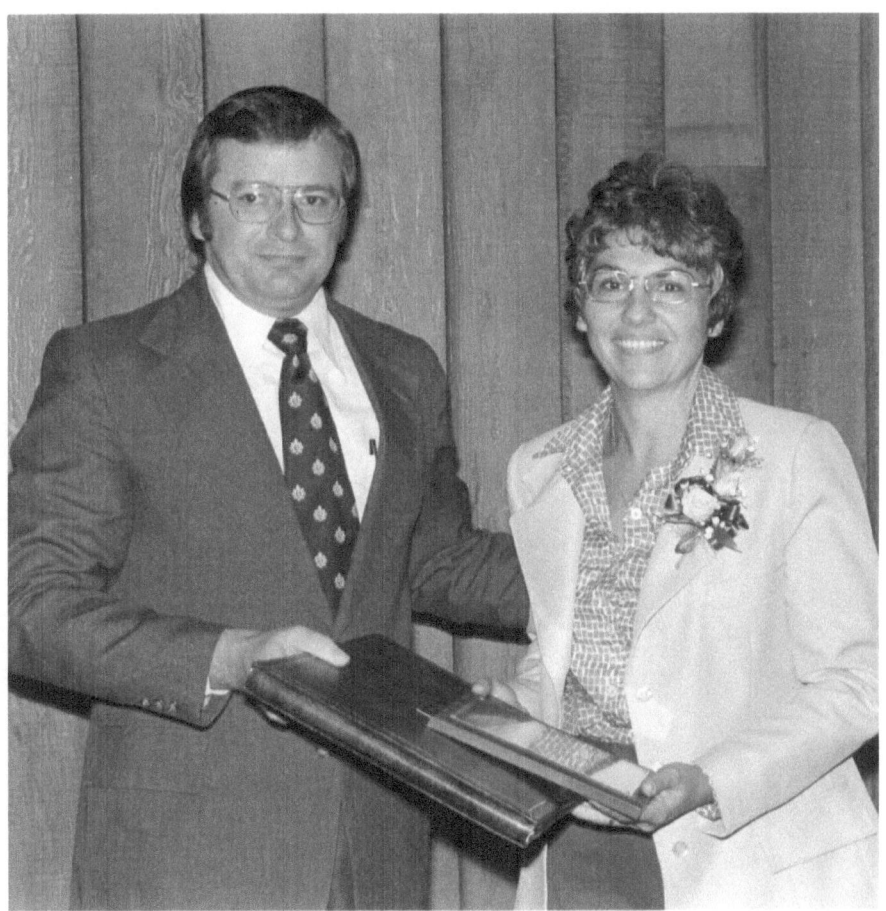

Terry Gets Award

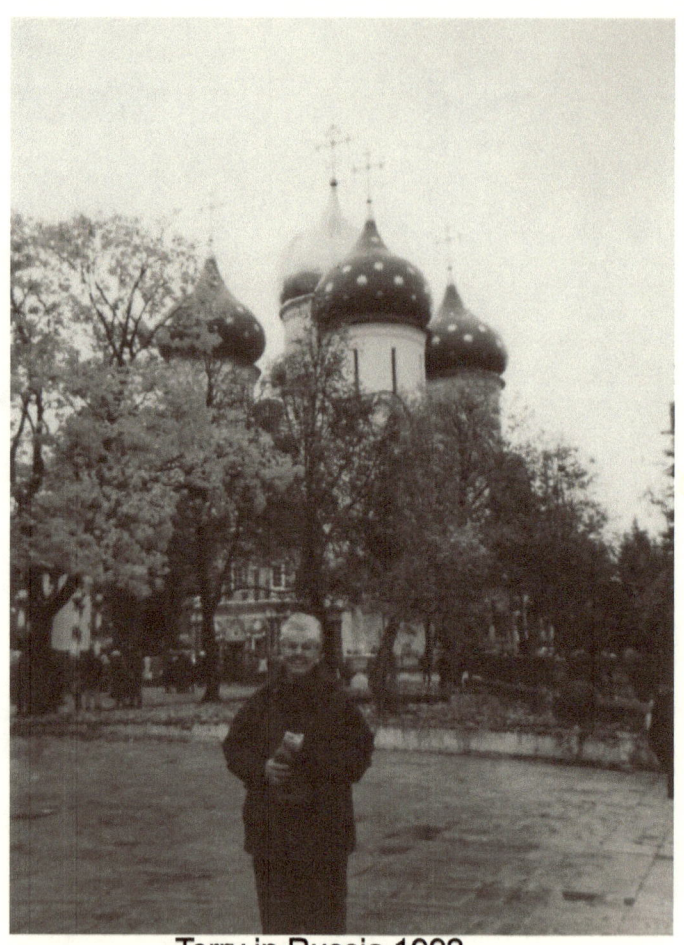

Terry in Russia 1992

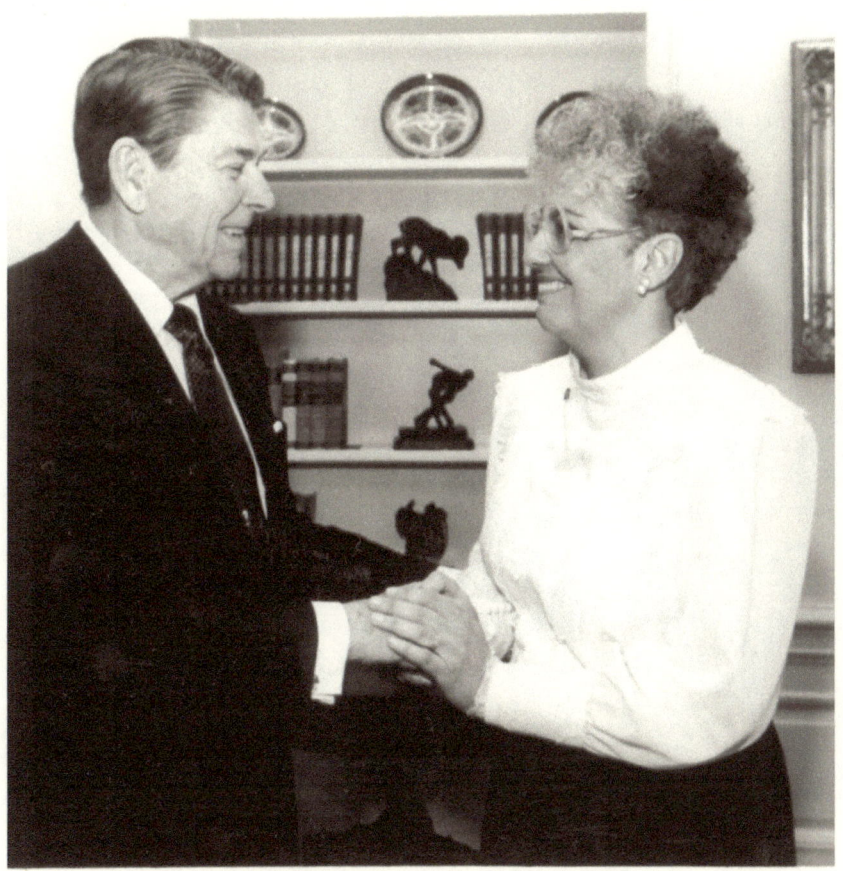

To Teresa Janora
With best wishes,
Ronald Reagan

Jan. 1988: Workers in the Field Prolife

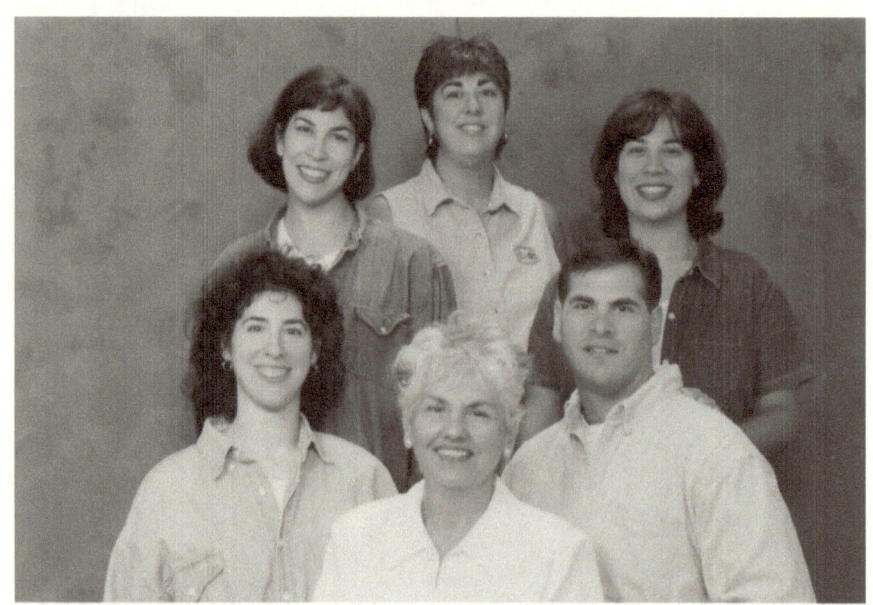

Terry's Children:Vicki, Serena, Lena, Joe, Tricia

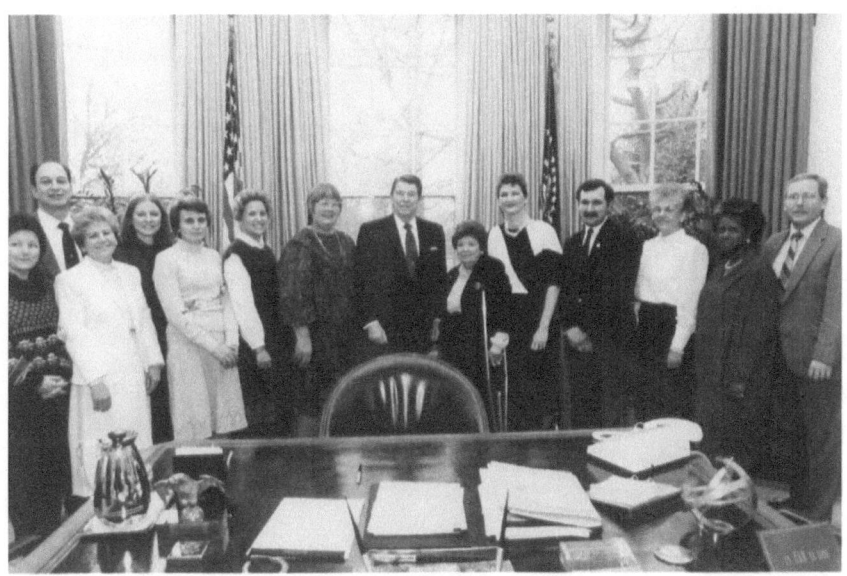

At the White House 1988

Chapter 4.

Terry's Story

Early Zeal

Thirty-five years ago, in 1972 I read an article in the Catholic Sentinel describing a new service whose purpose was to help women distressed by an untimely pregnancy. The group was in Portland. One photo of a woman seated opposite another woman with her back to the camera held my attention. The look of obvious tenderness and focused attention on the woman's face was unique.

I had five young children, which to me meant, experience in pregnancy. I thought helping a pregnant woman was a good idea. I went to Portland to see for myself. Bonnie Mannion, the director, gave me a concrete program to follow: 1) Get an office, 2) Get a phone 3) Buy pregnancy test kits. She was in touch with a woman who had founded a group called Birthright. Louise Summerhill, a Canadian, had realized in 1968 that abortion was coming to her country as it was already in the United States in California, Colorado and South Carolina and that a person-to-person, friendly, confidential and free service could be the means to offer desperate pregnant women an attractive alternative to abortion.

There were many people beginning to motivate the public to support pro-life efforts. One of them was Fr. John Powell, SJ. He wrote the book *Silent Holocaust*, in the early 1970s[4] and spent a year on sabbatical working for the pro-life cause by giving speeches and doing research.

---

[4] Paperback published by Argus in 1981: Powell, John, SJ. (1981). *The Silent Holocaust*. Allen, TX: Argus Communications.

He spoke in nearby Portland, Oregon, once and his perspective on the love which volunteers have for the mother and child was truly inspiring. He always praised our work

After two unsuccessful attempts to interest others in Eugene in the Birthright program a third meeting, after Roe v. Wade became law, brought many people. They were motivated to do something to counteract the Supreme Courts abortion decision. Things moved rapidly after that gathering. One pioneer of our local Eugene center was Marian Hodges, who used to bug me almost daily with telephone calls. I also gladly remember the support of Ellen Lyford, President of Right to Life, who acknowledged that though Marian was a gadfly, she did her work on me to get the center started and that was what mattered. Doris Storms and I met when she became president of Right to Life in 1976. She was a member of the local board along with Msgr. Edmund Murnane. Both were of great help in the beginning.

Frank McDonald, Director of St. Vincent de Paul was contacted. St. Vincent de Paul owned property a small, tiny really, one-room office. We rented it for $40.00 per month. A long flight of linoleum stairs led to our office. We were always afraid our pregnant women would slip and fall. We had a Board, including Msgr. Murnane, a staff, and an office. Thanks to Louise Summerhill and Denise Cocciolone of Birthright we had an ad copy and we placed ads in the Register Guard personals: *Pregnant? Need Help? Call 687-8651.* A letter of intent to charter was sent to Birthright headquarters in New Jersey. Everyone set to work studying the charter, painting and gathering furniture, and generally getting our office in order. The telephone number was obtained. Working off the volunteer sheet from the meeting, Sharin Mosnette and I made a staff list in shifts. On March 5, 1973, we opened a clean and freshly painted office. Our thanks to the Marist Brothers for the paint job and a filing cabinet. Fr. Vincent Coniff of St. Peters gave us chairs, which we still use, though they are reupholstered now. A desk and a typewriter were also donated. We were completely indebted to the kindness of others for all the office help and remain deeply grateful.

During this time we received and read a manuscript copy of *The Story of Birthright* (Summerhill, 1968). We also received a manual on how to answer the telephone from Birthright National USA. Our first Eugene director was Sharon Mosnette. However, after only five months of work her husband was transferred. I then became the Acting Director and have remained so to the writing of this book, with only some half dozen years where others assumed the task. Being Director is a consuming task, but has kept me focused on the needs of our office. The Director must be a role model to all of the volunteers. She must remain focused and never forget that every encounter with a client could be a life-changing event. She must care about her volunteers as in a family and let them know that they count in her eyes. None of us are professional counselors but rather wise, prudent friends. Prudence is key to directing an all volunteer office. Most of all, the Director must be a friend as is reflected in our ad motto: "Pregnant? Talk with a friend" and in our counseling philosophy.

A priest friend, Liam Cary, who wrote many speeches for me, characterized me as a woman of scarce personal resources. I humbly admit that he is right. I began this work with a meager knowledge of biology, personal counseling techniques and office personnel management. I also had no experience in fund raising, making budgets, or general business practices. I had to learn much about fetal development. I studied photos and read some basic biology books on development and brochures written by doctors. Many of these were very helpful, for example Dr. J.C. Wilke's (1971) *Abortion Questions and Answers* and the Italian brochure *Life, the First Miracle*, by Laura Barocchi (1977). My degrees in History, Political Science and Education were not of much help. On the job training was my only option. Thankfully other trained individuals helped teach me as well.

Despite the audacity of a program using solely volunteers, non-professional people to stem the tide of abortion, professional people were not lacking in our endeavor. Many of these professionals also felt the desire to help support life, and we provided the conduit to women in need. Dr. Sterling Ellsworth, a clinical psychologist, and later Lou Wagner who was studying counseling at the University of

Oregon, generously gave time and expertise in teaching me and other volunteers how to conduct an interview with a troubled woman. They gave us the questions to be asked and taught us the basic attitudes of a counselor. Lou was especially effective at teaching the volunteers.

Along with this expert help, a Sister of Social Service, Paula Vandegaer, produced videotapes on how to counsel and included the basic rules of confidentiality. Her work merits special recognition which I will discuss in greater detail later. Most importantly, she gave us a background on the history of crisis intervention and the knowledge that non-professionals are capable, if trained. She believed that ordinary people must help distressed women at this important time of decision. She was right and the pregnant mothers were attracted to the free, non-threatening program of simple friendship.

Over the years many like-minded professionals have blessed us with their talents and their belief in the suitability of this idea. The brochures produced by Pat Driscoll and her California group Womanity were great for educating young women. Other resources came from Eugene Kennedy and his book *Nuts and Bolts of Counseling*, and Dr. Greg Lester, a well respected Texas counselor.

People all over the USA were determined to push back against the abortion behemoth. Birthright was in the vanguard but professionals were willing to give us aid. This aid reminds me of the social reformers at the turn of the century. Many middle class educated women sought to meet the needs of poor women and their children and engaged in direct service through settlement houses and maternal childcare classes and also through charitable institutions, Hull House for one, but most especially those managed by nuns. These were successful in bringing humane treatment to children and mothers through the creation and staffing of their orphanages. The widespread desire to take care of mothers and children found expression and funding in charitable works like foundling hospitals, orphanages and later in the foster care home laws that protected women and children such as the Shephard Townshend Maternal and Child Welfare Act of 1921. This established a new mindset of caring for children in American society.

In the 1970s women came to Birthright in Eugene desperate for some help and guidance. Some were married women caught in extramarital affairs; at that time divorce was definitely not an option. Teens came, too, because at the time there were no school-based clinics, either. We had purchased life models, exact replicas of the pregnant uterus--and used them frequently to educate our clients. We found a few doctors willing to see our women for nothing. There were no full government insurance plans available in the 1970s for poor women. We filled a great need. Even so, we were still very naïve regarding office protocols. We would close our office and take the women in our cars to the doctors office, wait there, talk, and then take them back to our office. The women were supported, but the phone was left unmanned and all the while we wondered why our calls dropped off. Eventually we learned and improved and one volunteer always remained in the office to answer the phone. There were many simple lessons which we learned the hard way, but we carried on, because we knew we were meeting a need.

The Supreme Court had slyly couched its decision characterizing abortion as a private matter between the woman and her doctor. Therefore, our work in reaching into the pregnant woman's life could be viewed by society as interference or meddling. It reminds me of the concept of slavery, in that keeping of slaves was thought to be a situation outside of the concern of others. If you don't like slavery, don't keep slaves. Just don't interfere with those who do. Back off. While society's view on slavery has changed, this became the new perspective on abortion. This attitude made it difficult sometimes to enlist volunteer help. Yet deep in the human heart there is a basic understanding that a baby, no matter how small, is a precious God-given gift and that abortion is wrong. I used this concept when speaking at University of Oregon psychology classes by reading Dr. Seuss' *Horton Hears a Who*.[5] This was the motivation of our volunteers. It drove us out of our kitchens and into this new challenging arena. It drove us to organize ourselves into a working group with staff, office and advertising efforts. The horror of abortion on demand forced us to pour out our energies and to discover our

---

[5] Dr. Seuss. *Horton Hears a Who*. Random House, New York, 1954.

own strengths through our need to help others. And the women kept coming to our Birthright office. Among them were married, poor women, university of Oregon coeds and teens as well.

During this time (1973-1980) in addition to my work at the office, my family tried to offer a few pregnant women space in our own home. Most of these stays lasted for 2-3 days. It was so hard to see these women struggling. I will use substitute names for all the women I discuss. One young 16-year old pregnant girl, I'll call her Jenny, we picked up in front of her home because her mom threw her out. Her boxes were on the sidewalk, on top a teddy bear. Jenny stayed with us for weeks sharing a bedroom with the older girls. We even got her a place in the Catholic high school. We grew to love her but eventually her mom called her and insisted she return home. Her mother said that all would be forgiven. Unfortunately, Jenny was forced into a late abortion (saline). The mother came to my house and threatened me, so we lost contact. Years later Jenny called me; we met and talked a bit. She was a mother to two children but her home life was a shambles. When we arranged to meet again, she had disappeared from her place of work. I still think of her a beautiful girl--young, burdened by many sorrows.

So intense was my desire to share the work of my fellow Birthright workers that during family cross-country trips, when we got the family settled in a motel I'd get the local yellow pages phone book and look up the Birthright office. I'd call the next day and have a nice chat with the telephone volunteer, sometimes even talking to the office director. It was a thrilling and enriching experience for me to get to talk over the same problems and ideas and exchange tips. Sometimes if it wasn't too out of the way, we would pass by the local office on our way to our next destination.

In the early days many of us attended our clients births. I remember one special girl, one of our first clients. Pam was a teen whose mother was so furious about her pregnancy that she threatened to turn her out of the home. Pam called me when she was in labor. I stayed with her at the hospital. I remember she was so brave, never uttered a word during labor. She sat cross-legged, yoga-style, and had an amazingly peaceful birth. We kept in touch for years.

I was amazed and so edified by the bravery of the pregnant women I met at my office. I myself did not appreciate being pregnant. I didn't like the discomfort, ill feelings, pain, etc. I was frightened, too. But these women, many against great unhappiness and sorrow over the lack of home and parents, evil treatment by boyfriends, kept going despite obvious morning sickness and poverty to deliver their babies. Ina May Gaskin (1975), in *Spiritual Midwifery* gives a beautiful, encouraging vision of birth. Unborn babies, in their turn, profoundly influence their mothers.[6]

The decade of the 1980s was one of building our reputation of helping many women. Our pregnancy test was still a slide that one had to rock back and forth to get a positive or negative result. It was difficult to read but home tests, even though on the market, were very poor quality, inaccurate, difficult to read and expensive. We were needed. Free tests and free clothing were always in demand and we ran 90-100 tests per month.

Our office moved three times before October 1998 when we finally moved our office to the present location, across from Planned Parenthood, and the next year a donor covered the entire cost of an ultrasound machine. The ultrasound technician from an OB/GYN office came every other week to oversee our techs. It seemed as though the dream and prediction of Dr. Nathanson (1981) for a "window to the womb" that would save unborn had come true!

Our endeavor to open a Eugene office began with the inspiration of a simple article in the Catholic Sentinel and the example of a center in Portland. With the help of Birthright the vision was watered with our zeal to serve and so has succeeded. The Eugene office became a reality and continued to grow into a place of shelter, making a difference for many victims of the abortion culture.

---

[6] *Spiritual Midwifery* first published in 1975 and then again in 1977, 1980, 1990, and 2002.

Duties and Challenges Related to the Office of Regional Consultant

In addition to directing the Eugene Birthright office I was appointed Regional Consultant, (RC) in 1976. In my job as RC I had to plan and coordinate meetings for the Northwest and beyond. Sometimes it required flying to centers to give workshops, other times I could drive. Always, I learned and gained so much from contact with other pro-life women. "I can do all things in Him who strengthens me," comes to mind looking back. When I began this new position I wrote to my fellow consultants and received some guidance. One unforgettable letter from Marie Hughes of Santa Rosa, CA, shocked and even scared me! Her analogy for pro-lifers was that of trying to make a group of unruly horses become a team. Perhaps this should not be so surprising. United in our desire to help, each office was locally shaped and influenced by the style of the leaders and volunteers who ran it. We stood up for what we knew was right, but we were still all human, with our varied strengths and weaknesses. As a rule pro-lifers do not go with the flow.

When I visited the regional centers I found that some of the directors wanted to be exempted from keeping regular hours for their offices. They wanted to answer the phones from home and didn't see a need for regular attendance at regional meetings or at a local office. Some wanted to prevent abortion through abstinence counseling or presenting Natural Family Planning (NFP). It was frustrating for me. It was my job to direct everyone in accordance with the Birthright charter and to share the hard lessons we had already acquired but I greatly disliked having to correct adult women. Counseling on abstinence and NFP, though very valuable are outside our mission, and would be essentially impossible in our clients unstable, transitory relationships. I used the telephone to keep in touch and I wrote a newsletter for the NW region. It was impossible to be aware of everything, though. Early on one woman deceived me into thinking she was still the Director. It was several months later that I found out she had been replaced by her Board. The strength of each office Director was clearly of critical importance. I could see that the weakness of a Director might lead to Board decisions not in keeping with the Birthright vision. The difficulty of having all volunteers was summed up concisely by Dr. LeRoy Thompson, Jr. in his book, *Mastering the Challenges of Change (1994)*: "How challenging it is to have to motivate volunteers over whom you have hardly any authority but who have a tremendous bearing and impact on the success of the organization."

Some directors found it hard to recruit because of the nature of the work. I had to agree with them it was dirty business, knowing about the procedure and all the attendant deadly ways people used poor panicky women to make money. Many underhanded practices were going on such as selling baby parts - skin, liver, brain - to beauty care manufacturers. Abortion doctors and middlemen were preying on the sick/vain to promise better skin for a new lease on life from the unborn baby (Crutcher, 1996). Even so, I eventually found that acting as director was the niche I was meant to occupy, in spite of the challenges.

Shooting Stars: The Volunteers

Many wonderful and committed women stepped up to the challenge of volunteering. Yet in spite of all that these volunteers desired to do, many were unable to follow through on the entirety of their plans. Some would promise to do a project that was desperately needed. They would present their plan to go to area churches to advertise and recruit others and or get needed dollars. Unfortunately, often before the project would get rolling, they would disappear in the flow of their own lives. Perhaps they would find another job, or their husband was transferred, or lost his job. Sometimes they became pregnant, or just left for other endeavors. Nevertheless, every volunteer has added an important ingredient in some way: creating ads, reupholstering furniture, suggesting new office procedures, or just sharing ideas, ideals, and thoughts. I will be forever grateful to all of them. I have tried to enlist the help of some veteran staff to train others, but in general they cannot because of commitments. I regard volunteers as meteors in the night sky, brilliant lights that flash across the darkness and disappear. There is one that is even helping me by typing these notes! God be praised. For many years there has emerged a wonderful consoling team spirit wherein the staff has caught the vision of helping the pregnant woman in a most focused way.

Some volunteers who came to our office to help out revealed to me that they were victims of abortions themselves. They were truly bereft of any help because their professional counselors tended to neglect the past abortion, delving into childhood issues instead and completely missing the fact that the abortion was the cause of their depression and anxiety. So many different women have volunteered. There have been hundreds during these 35 years, young, mature, married. Some, like Agnes with her brood of 9 and Mary with 10, had many children and grandchildren. Others were newly married, college girls from the University of Oregon, or even college men. We have welcomed a football player, a would-be counselor in training, even a husband and wife team. Some stayed as volunteers for years, like Cindy, a can do worker who was with us for about 10 years, Juanita and Fernie for 17 years, Susan and Lee for 20 years and Lucy who is still here after 35 years. We have grown up together. Lucy and I had very young children in the beginning. Lucy had a new baby during part of her term as Director. Marriages, deaths, baptisms, births, parental care, children, new ventures, promotions for husbands, transfers, were all part of our lives as staff people. As Louise used to say in Birthright, the volunteers are the staff.

Some volunteers cannot come to the office but help out as consultants, especially for Spanish language clients. When there is a Spanish speaker at the office now we rejoice. Being able to talk frankly and in-depth to a woman about her problem pregnancy is crucial to providing all the help we can through our office.

It was depressing that some pro-life people scoffed at our efforts to prevent abortion. One doctor said to me, "you have a tiger by the tail." These discouraging words as well as my constant talk on the telephone and the feeling of abandoning my own children produced constant nagging thoughts. Peers would engage me in conversations saying that they preferred to care for their own children rather than trying to help others. Charity begins at home, they would repeat to me. But I kept going and some volunteers stayed on for years with me and with the women we helped. This is the charity we were called to and we really got to know and love each other as we worked together.

After the initial interview and appointment with a client we would often call upon the Carmelite nuns on Greenhill Rd. to pray in particular for one woman or another. The Carmelites have been and remain valued partners in our work. We rely on their prayer support and wisdom to keep us, the volunteers, going at the office as well. They are always ready with an encouraging word and love.

In many ways the volunteers have trained me. The difficulty of being a manager of an all-volunteer staff means dealing with the constant coming and going of volunteers and the repeat training sessions. Rarely would I have the luxury of having a veteran volunteer on the shift with a new one to do training. This change of staff has caused me to want to run away sometimes. Over the years I have needed to hear the words of the wiser volunteers who would watch our clients and say, "There but for the grace of God go I." They would even marvel at how together our girls were despite their awful circumstances at home. This kind of insight has humbled me and helped me to appreciate our clients in their distressing disguises. It is amazing to ponder that this attitude of love and acceptance in action is truly the prevailing attitude of most of the 1st Way/Birthright volunteers and this made for heaven on earth for me.

By working to offer alternatives to abortion, we, the grass roots volunteers, stepped into a new cultural divide without knowing it. As Anne Hendershott put it, the two Americas, are not the one recently described by John Edwards of race and class, but, those who believe that the lives of the unborn must be protected and the other America (that) thinks all women should have access to abortion on demand no matter how late in the pregnancy (Hendershott, 2006). The volunteers have focused on the trees, rather than the forest, and worked to meet each client where she was.

About Our Clients

Our society, and in particular modern radical feminism, is averse to the idea of powerlessness in women. Abortion is said to give women power over their bodies. I learned that individual women don't live out this nice-sounding ideal. For most of them there was a victimhood as pregnant women. They felt a certain resignation and desperation towards their men. This was understandable to me being brought up in an old school Italian home where papa ruled the roost. The powerlessness of women was not a foreign aspect. I could sympathize with the worldview of these women. Actually, science and psychology bear out this attitude of pregnancy as well. Pregnancy hormones increase the feelings of dependence on the mothers partner, giving greater weight to his desires and opinions. From an evolutionary perspective, pregnant women need the support of their partner and their community to perpetuate the species, particularly as her ability to gather food and supply her own needs diminishes through the pregnancy (Matthews-Green, 1981).

Some clients had attitudes and backgrounds completely outside of my middle class existence. They were singularly without dreams or even expectations for their future. Single, poor, from disconnected families, their relationships with boyfriends were usually transitory. Yes, most emphatically, they wanted the boyfriends attention and approval even if it meant having the abortion they did not want. They were vulnerable in a way that I had not seen up close. Of course all girls are vulnerable to boyfriends. I can speak from my own youthful emotions, but these girls were different. All but a few put up a front when receiving the pregnancy test result. When the test comes out positive and as elated as they are, if a boyfriend or mom said no, they would get an abortion. Any negative reaction would send them to the abortionist. Worse, some Moms would threaten to drive the young girl out of the home. And sadder still, sometimes there was no parent; the girl was living on the street or under a bridge. One volunteer reported that while she was riding on the bus, a young mom stood at the front holding out her young baby and said Who wants him? She cried and then sat down. The struggles of women who are presented with the awful choice of killing their child cannot be overstated. The depressing lack of support that they receive from the people closest to them only makes the situation more overwhelming. *The Corner*, by David Simon and Edward Burns offers a good description of this depressed viewpoint.

Many of our girls lacked the supportive relationships necessary to pursue the desire of their own hearts. Chris came to 1st Way for a pregnancy test. She was a young woman living with her boyfriend at his family's home with the family's approval and support. Her own mom lived in a distant city and was in an unstable situation. When Chris test came up positive, she was horrified but told the counselor she was sure her boyfriend and his family would be OK with it. After telephoning Chris, the counselor was told that it was not OK because her would be mother-in-law thought the baby would hurt the future plans of her son. During this interim a donor provided $1,000.00 to be given to a pregnant woman who desired to further her education. Chris was asked to come to the office to talk and both together searched out programs adapted to her situation (GED) and also apartments that she could afford because of the obvious fact that if she did not abort she would be out of her home. Opportunities were found all that remained was for Chris to announce her departure. Instead, when the volunteer called Chris to arrange transportation, no one answered the phone. A few hours later, the boyfriends mother called to tell the volunteer that they had returned from the abortion procedure in Portland. She was tearful but wanted to know if they could still have the $1,000.00.

One volunteer received a call from Anna. She was 32 years old and living in a Women Space shelter because she was fleeing a physically abusive boyfriend. Anna had two children, a boy of 14 and a girl of 11. She called First Way because she thought we did abortions. The volunteer asked her to come in for a pregnancy test just to make sure she was pregnant. She came in for her appointment that day and they had a very long, heart-to-heart talk. She was 32, had no job and, as I indicated, was fleeing an abusive boyfriend. The volunteer called First Place Family Center and gave her a referral to them for any help that they could provide her. An ultrasound appointment was made for her for the next day. When she left we hoped and prayed that she would show up for the US but the next day, she did not show. She was in a terrible situation and we are convinced that she went ahead with the abortion. When the volunteer tried to reach her later, her cell phone had been disconnected. She had told us that it might be because her boyfriend paid the bill. We learn many things at First Way. We learn that we cannot save all of the babies. We learn that we cannot improve the living circumstances for all of the mothers and children with whom we come in contact. But above all, we learn not to judge women who make the terribly difficult decision to abort their babies. Many of them are in extremely complicated situations like Anna's. We know that God will be merciful.

Tragically, Christy Wedmore, a community social worker for the Lane County Public Health Department, indicates that there are poor results for pregnant women in the Eugene community. There is a lack of access to health care, but also distrust of the medical community, poor nutrition, and methamphetamine addiction (Staff Meeting Notes, March 2006).

Who can say these women are independent and free in their decisions. Abortion or not, they are in desperate need of a love that places no demands and a friendship that values their innate humanity. This is the foundation of our work, to offer that love and to be that friend. Pregnant women and mothers are not meant to be alone. These are the facts that must remain in the forefront in recalling the story of our movement.

Counseling

How could one approach a woman in crisis without becoming emotional or detached in a cold way? This is a great challenge. We all wanted to prevent the abortion. The staff knew the facts, had seen so many movies or diagrams or pictures of abortions but how does one convey this data without being emotional and instead remaining calm and loving. The abortion education part of the interview where we have to explain the details of abortion took some courage for all the volunteers, me included, to be clear and up front without an emotional overlay. The Holy Father made the following remarks in a Wednesday General Audience (translation 2008) regarding St. Peter's own struggles with truly understanding the mission of Christ and his journey to full conversion as described in Mark chapter 8:

> I think that these different conversions of St. Peter and his whole figure are a motive of great consolation and a great teaching for us. We also desire God, we also want to be generous, but we also expect God to be strong in the world and that he transform the world immediately, according to our ideas and the needs we see.

God opts for another way. God chooses the way of transformation of hearts in suffering and humility. And we, like Peter, must always be converted again. We must follow Jesus and not precede Him. He shows us the way. Peter tells us: "You think you have the recipe and that you have to transform Christianity, but the Lord is the one who knows the way. It is the Lord who says to me, who says to you, 'Follow me!' And we must have the courage and humility to follow Jesus, as He is the Way, the Truth and the Life."[7]

This quote is very relevant to our work as volunteer counselors. We learned all that we could, but in the end counseling women is about loving the mother and child and getting out of God's way as He speaks to them through us. Please do not misunderstand. We never proselytize or witness to these women. Rather we strive to be the vehicle that Christ can work through in their lives; the good neighbor who feeds the hungry and clothes the naked. With our actions we say, "You are of value to us!"

As I mentioned previously, we were blessed with early training in counseling from Dr. Sterling Ellsworth and the videotapes produced by Paula Vandegaer as we began our office in Eugene. Another great help has been the Motivational Interview training by Linda Keepers

---

[7] Pope Benedict XVI. General Audience, May 17, 2006. Translated by Zenit.org, Vatican City.

of Christians Addressing Family Abuse (CAFA). We have been taught how to be with the client, on her side, as well as various client attitudes, and how to take her part and build her up.

Lou Wagner offered more counseling experience and education to volunteers. Among regular meetings, his training was one of the very best presented and attended by volunteers. With better training we were able to impact more pregnant women and to successfully encourage them in carrying their babies to term. It was through Lou's guidance that we had a substantial list of procedures on how to work one-on-one work with our women. These included many basics of counseling including active listening, body position, non-verbal communication, and eye contact.

Father M. Mannion was usually part of the National Life Center (NLC) Birthright convention program. He presented inspiring talks regarding women he counseled, his experiences with past abortions, and our need for compassion and understanding. His talks and his book, *Abortion and Healing: a Cry to Be Whole* (Mannion, 1996), have also helped improve our counseling abilities.

The counseling we learned to give was not like that which is usually paid for with a professional. If there is one word to sum up and describe crisis pregnancy counseling such as 1st Way offers, it is this, personal. Some of the stories of our girls show the difference that this makes.

Phyllis, a new 1st Way volunteer, talked at length to Cindy who wanted an abortion because the father of the baby was an illegal alien. When Cindy did not show for her ultrasound, Phyllis was called by the ultrasound technician. Phyllis came in to the office. She called Cindy to encourage her to come in for an ultrasound. Cindy consented, and although it was not her shift, Phyllis stayed with her through the ultrasound. Because of the ultrasound pictures and the friendship of Phyllis, Cindy changed her mind about the abortion.

Lacey came to 1st Way because she needed our confirmation of pregnancy so that she could get on the Oregon Health Plan. Anita was the volunteer who met here for that first visit. Anita continued to call her after her appointment was concluded and found out that Lacey needed a ride to her doctor appointment. Anita helped her get the ride and invited Lacey to lunch. In the course of time Anita found out that Lacey was desperate for a means to pay her rent. Her boyfriend worked at a very low paying job. Anita not only found a good job for her but also found an agency that would pay her rent until she got on her feet. Anita was a counselor and so much more, because she allowed her relationship with Lacey to be personal. One volunteer, touching one life at a time, that is success in our work.

As Director I sometimes found local speakers who offered us assistance in continuing to improve our methods through the years. One such find was Jack Harrington, a counselor for the 4J School District in Eugene. Although never involved in pro-life work of any sort, he grasped the vision of what volunteer workers must be for the pregnant woman. Through his suggestions, we transformed the office itself. We rearranged furniture to his specifications. The two sofa love seats were placed facing each other, we gathered life-giving images (a pregnant woman and baby, a family Mom, Dad with baby). We had artwork of pregnant women in silhouette, original portrait of a newborn, etc. We changed our initial encounter by presenting to the woman, in ourselves, a person eager to invite her into our office as a friend to give her tea and cookies and ask her to fill out a brief questionnaire so we could get to know her better and what her needs might be.[8]

Jack introduced us to the idea of writing down the woman's every thought regarding the pregnancy and he called it Force Field. We would draw a line down the center of a paper so that the mother could list everything good and bad about this pregnancy on the two sides. He taught us not to be afraid of what she would say negatively about the pregnancy, to be calm, accepting of her desires and outlook. This left us detached in one way but able to see in the Good/Bad list a way to share her thoughts. Using that list, listening to her, we might help her to look kindly on a pregnancy. Some day in the future when

---

[8] Due to changes in attitudes in recent years, we have been led to modify our baby displays for more neutral settings. We are still weighing this change.

things were right, even now with this one too, she might go to term because of our help and care.

Contrary to some perspectives, volunteers can be the very best counselors, because they can be present outside of a rigid schedule. They are free to make the relationship personal. Volunteers can work on a day off, they can give home phone numbers, and they can visit and stand along side the pregnant women through and beyond the birth of their child. This is the support a good friend would give. Just this week when Sandy called, a volunteer was able to encourage her to call her doctor back for an explanation of what was said to her as a passing comment regarding her baby and his position in her uterus. This is counseling made personal.

Travels and Meetings: National and International

Some of the work of running a CPC did not involve direct client contact. There were also plenty of opportunities for travel as a Regional Consultant. These trips sometimes allowed us to support others, and sometimes offered support to us. In 1988 I was one of ten Birthright Regional Consultants to meet President Reagan along with some dozen pro-lifers engaged in diverse pro-life work. It was all so exciting, entering the oval office one at a time, greeted by President Reagan. Secret service men were stationed around the room. I really didn't hear much of what Reagan said but I knew it was complimentary of our work in the field. I concentrated instead on soaking up the room decor and atmosphere. A fitting home for my country, I thought.

In 1992, I accompanied Denise to a conference in Kaunas, Lithuania, and Moscow, Russia. We were to deliver messages in both places. The sacrificial generosity of our Lithuanian and Russian hosts during that same conference was truly remarkable. One of our hostesses gave us lunch in her tiny apartment in a huge apartment complex. I remember the elevators were broken. We walked up seven flights. There were no cupboards for her dishes, no refrigerator and seven of us sat at her kitchen table while she served us a hearty meal. Her stove was a propane outdoor grill. We could only guess that she must have spent her scarce cash for us, her guests. Later, at the high school where our talk was presented on how a Birthright office works, several women came up to tell us of their abortions. Some had 15-20 during their lifetimes.

In Moscow I also had the honor of meeting Dr. Jerome Lejeune. He is truly a humble man though a scientific giant. I have recently learned how much more he did for the cause of life. In fact Pope John Paul II appointed him as president of the Pontifical Academy for Life shortly before his death. in 1994. In fact, the promotion of a cause for his canonization began in 2007. The memory of just his gentle presence remains with me to this day. His testimony regarding the individuality of human embryos in a domestic relations case, Davis v Davis, was enlightening.[9]

We spoke to large crowds, more than one thousand in a university auditorium in Lithuania. In Moscow, Russia it was a smaller venue, mostly doctors and nurses. In Lithuania we stayed at people's homes and apartments. I remember being so cold but our hostess was so kind, giving us animal skins for covers. I accompanied her to shop and saw that there was practically nothing in this small local convenience store. There were 4-5 bottles of milk and small cakes, the rest were bare shelves. Some of the participants acted as tour guides after the presentation and they were full of information regarding soldiers taking over the churches to stable their horses. It seemed so hard for them to imagine people volunteering, While in their neighborhoods Moms were compelled to place their children in learning centers while they worked all day.

In 1995 Denise asked me to attend the Vatican Conference on the Family in October of that year. The conference was headed by Bishop Elio Sgreccia and Cardinal Lopez Trujillo. There were three days of formal talks with language translations for each speaker in the general assembly and then breakout groups in our language.

---

[9] Tennessee Circuit Court for Blount Co. Davis v King, Seven Frozen Embryos. Case No E-14496, 1989. Blount Co, Tennessee.

Listening to the people who came from all over the world and then being able to personally talk with those English speakers from Australia, Cameroon, England, Scotland, Zimbabwe, Molowi, was a wonderful experience. There were study groups for Evangelum Vitae. Pope John Paul II even gave a brief audience for us participants.

I met some Italian women towards the end of the conference, whom later I was invited to visit in 1999 in Viareggio, Italy. They headed up the CAVs, Centri Auito Alla Vita. Theirs was a combination of social work, food distribution and pregnancy counseling. Their office was attached to a room in the same building that provided free lunches to the poor.

Workers at the Pregnancy Care Center wrote an open letter to John Paul II, published in a pro-life magazine. In regards to their work they said that Providence assists us and accompanies us in the battle that often overwhelms our own struggle. The workers know that the attitude of pregnant women will certainly determine the destiny of the human race. Moreover, they have also said that helping a woman to find her true self, helping her understand the joy of being the guardian of such a gift, is an awesome task. I also very much appreciated their philosophy that there can be no competition between mother and baby: to save the life of the baby is to build up the happiness of the mother.

The Holy Father, in his turn, called the CAV workers "the people of life." I also visited the main CAV on Via Scipioni in Rome in 1992 which housed a combination pregnancy care center, educational center in one building. CAVs even today, continue to give financial aid to pregnant women from their sustenance. They do not depend on the State of Italy but each volunteer is assessed between 25-50 Euros per month along with the time spent at their offices to aid the work.

There is a broad network of support for life in Italy. The CAVs operate a national phone line, the equivalent of an American 1-800 phone number, called a green number, SOSVITA. Project Gemma gives material aid to help a pregnant woman up to 18 months after the birth of her child. Other assistance offered to Italian women include a section of Avvenire, an official Catholic newspaper titled *Life Issues* and a weekly radio program called "Yes to Life." "Agata Smeralda" supports orphanages in Brazil by monthly contributions to encourage authors and editors to create works that promote the culture of life. There is a prize given yearly by another related group, the New Life Foundation.

The activities of the CAVs "are not social work, nor an expression of sentimentality, nor simply information in the sense of psychiatric consultation. The workers at CAVs help the other person to make her own personal choice; the most suitable to her particular situation. Just as we strive for here in the US, they listen respectfully so that they can enter into a relationship with another who is in possession of her own rights and not an object of pity. In addition, there is guaranteed anonymity and respect for the mother who has shown the strength to give birth to a new life" (Cassini, 1974).

Such travels sound almost glamorous now, yet the purpose and the heart of every one of the journeys was women and children. Human life is valued around the world and knowing this reinforced my will to continue when the work was especially difficult. Hopefully it supported those we visited as well.

National conventions were closer to home, yet still difficult to reach and costly. Even so they were infinitely valuable for sharing knowledge and uniting the members of the movement. I so enjoyed the meetings, conferences, and staff meetings. I found that others were experiencing the same scenes of abortion horror but were still working, sharing and laughing, enjoying and relishing their lives and families, and I was gaining insight into how others presented themselves and their offices. I met very zealous, intelligent women and men from Eugene to Africa and Europe to Canada.

From time to time we would be lucky enough to receive some professional help for ourselves in the trenches. At a convention or meeting, a thought-provoking program would refresh our flagging spirits. One such experience occurred at one of our regular yearly meetings. Instead of the usual instruction from an obstetrician on fetal development, PhD counseling tips, or an ad person on the latest marketing ploy, Sally Carr, RN, the Regional Consultant for Utah, presented us with a series of questions. These questions (for example, What is your biggest challenge, what do you struggle with most) were to be answered on large white 5x8 cards and then shared with the group. This exercise helped us to open our hearts to one another regarding the struggles for time, self-doubt, small client loads, ignorance or disregard for the preciousness of life, amorality, client bias against adoption, lack of shelter homes, and welfare obstacles. On that day sharing these challenges with others at that meeting was more helpful to keeping our work going than any technical information would have been. Sally also shared with us her remarkable instinctive approach to women in crisis. She was also a nurse and became one of the wise counselor models for me.

Again at conferences we benefited greatly from many technical speakers as well. Jean Stacker Garton, helped us learn how to frame the issues in more realistic and honest terms. As author of *Who Broke the Baby?* (Garton, 1979) and a speaker at a conference, she alerted us to the importance of word choice when referring to our topics: Baby, not blob or fetus; Abortion, not the procedure, or choice or termination, etc. She exposed the falsehood of slogans like "every child a wanted child," and shared how the abortion industry tries to obscure the truthfulness of what happens in an abortion. Correct/accurate language is vitally important to helping a woman know the truth.

Another tremendous insight into the difficulties that our clients faced when deciding whether to undergo abortion was made clear in Frederica Mathews-Greens (1994) book, *Real Choices.* Hers was the first extensive survey of women who had undergone abortions and the complex reasons why they felt compelled to seek abortion. A very useful part of her book deals with some positive options and proposals that pregnancy care workers could and do offer to clients. For example, sincerely offering of our friendship, holding a positive view of marriage to the baby's father, viewing adoption (especially open adoption) as a viable and noble choice, and sharing employment plans that do not include welfare as a permanent situation allows the client to see all of her options as real plausible possibilities for achieving a new productive future.

I met Herb Ratner, MD at an early Birthright convention. He published many studies on maternal care, breast-feeding, and a whole culture of life and love, birth etc. I found these works very helpful in understanding the big picture of how mothering and children impact our culture. This helped me engage in discussing the positive sides of choosing to give an unborn child the chance at life.

Fr. Michael Mannion, now Msgr., Board Member of NLC, was another person who opened the door to understanding and loving our clients through his first hand experience with post-abortive women. His book, *Abortion and Healing: A Cry to be Whole (1996),* Mannion provided a vision of true healing that we could initiate at the time of our clients visit to the office. He especially insists that we should encourage bonding to the new child for the post-abortive woman. This is accomplished , in part, by listening to her story of her previous abortion. There can be no bonding without first healing the past, he said. Another speaker, counselor Eileen Curro says that asking about her abortion we get only a piece of the woman when she comes to our office, but its an essential step towards her ultimate healing.

Conference speakers like Fr. Mike Mannion, Olivia Gans, Drs. Philip Ney and Vincent Rue, Ellen Curro and Vickie Thorn were among others who impressed upon all the volunteers that the wounds our women were enduring because of their abortions affected all their decisions. It was, indeed, a challenge to redirect our counseling to bring out and acknowledge grief and guide the women towards needed healing through referrals to Rachel's Vineyard, in addition to dealing with current pregnancies. In the first 30 years there was no support for mothers grieving after an abortion. Rachel's Vineyard is now a very valuable tool for helping these women.

The traveling that I was able to do and the conferences that the Directors and Regional Consultants attended may seem in some ways frivolous to the grass roots work that we had committed ourselves to doing. Yet looking back at how much those events taught, refreshed and sustained me in the journey, I realize that it was crucial to know that one was not working alone, but was a part of a much wider network.

Speaking Engagements as Local Director

A few teachers at local schools, in particular Springfield High School, and some in Eugene, invited me to speak to students in the early years. I took life models and did a presentation on the services of Birthright. I liked to speak on the three necessary elements of a good decision and how they apply to the decision of whether to abort a child: 1. Facts (prenatal), 2. Options (parenting and adoption, since abortion they already knew about) and 3. Support (of reliable friends such as Birthright.) I believe that these talks offered some clarity for high school students facing any decision. I would give a hypothetical case, a stick figure on the blackboard and give out how Birthright helped in every single situation. It was a daunting task and I would return to my home and family very tired. Amazingly, I hardly know how I managed to make dinner and return to just being Mom in the evenings.

However, in general in the local public high schools it was evident that the teachers were not at all pro-life. I remember a movie shown during class. It included a scene where Bishops with their miters on, were processing in a cathedral maybe St. Peters in Rome and a voiceover saying that some people, especially the Catholic Church was rigid and wanted to control the lives of all people. Imagine how that statement went over with teens. A balanced presentation was clearly needed. Adoption agencies were loath to come to high schools to explain services. Lately there has been a change in that stance. Agencies have produced videos like *A Special Kind of Love*, and *A Sensible Choice*. These videos are a great help to pregnancy centers counseling women on the positive aspects of adoption.

Locally in Eugene I was disappointed and shocked to see how entrenched the culture of death had quickly become. My children were taught biology by Mary Gossert Wedoff at a Catholic school.

She was later a top speaker and advocate for Planned Parenthood. Her mentor was Sol Gordon. Sol wrote and spoke about being a hip parent through his pamphlets called teachable moments on sex education. He is now a noted author on the subject.[Gordon] Even as a parent I was not granted a hearing in Mary Gossert Wedoff's class. On one of my speaking engagements at the Junior High School in Springfield, I was allowed to sit in on the Planned Parenthood presentation. It was only because another mother of a student was also present that we were granted the right to hear. Abstinence was briefly mentioned but was dismissed as practically impossible to attain and so safe sex through condom use or other means, mostly the pill, was presented.

Once I received an invitation from a University of Oregon professor, Ed Kime, to speak to his psychology class. I took the book my children were reading, *Horton Hears a Who* (Seuss, 1954). It seemed very appropriate. I don't know if I made any impact on his class. He never asked me back. But, I noticed that theme, A person's a person, no matter how small, has been used more recently in some pro-life materials such as bumper stickers.

I have not been invited into any classrooms in recent years, though I also have not approached the schools myself. There is a greater emphasis now on abstinence education which would not be the type of talk that I could offer. This spring, however, I had the opportunity to participate in our local Right to Life Conference. I presented some background and history of the grass roots CPC movement while Karen Tameling, executive director of the Options CPC in Corvallis, presented the current methods used at the CPC. Speaking engagements are tiring for me now, but it is still good to be able to share our work whenever possible.

Abortion the Great Evil: Moving Forward

Discouragement. It is a natural response to the 50 million abortions that have occurred since Roe v. Wade. So many millions of children. It is an ugly battle which no one wants to dwell upon for long. The numbers of successes are so few in comparison to the lives lost. It is hard to remember that God does not necessarily measure success in numbers and statistics. As Blessed Teresa of Calcutta has said, We are not called to be successful, but to be faithful. That is the goal.

In the face of this great evil, I have often felt alone and rarely been confident in my work. During a particular time of trial, I learned the Serenity Prayer. It gave me peace as I struggled with strong feelings of incompetence. The Carmelite nuns have been a spiritual example for me. The Carmelite Way of Life gave me more structure in my prayer life and greater peace. I am now a lay member of the Carmelites for eight years and so continue to participate in the Liturgy of the Hours and meditation.

The death of my mother increased my feelings of aloneness. My mother was always very supportive of my work. As a child I remember how very considerate she was of pregnant women. She was very aware of who was pregnant--friends, acquaintances or even people we would pass by on the street or subway, etc. She wanted them to have seats on the train or bus and she would tell me to give up my own seat for them. When she knew of a woman in labor I knew she was thinking of them during their "time." During my labors she was so concerned and "felt the pains" along with me. Mom's inspiration has helped me in my endeavors, working in a grassroots movement with an all-volunteer staff.

One way I used to keep steadily at the work of attending to my CPC in spite of my feelings of inadequacy was to read something everyday about abortion: descriptions of techniques, for example, exposés of Planned Parenthood, partial birth or something in the news regarding legislation, congressional hearings, really anything about abortion, even just 10 minutes but something specifically regarding abortion. And, information was never difficult to find, always available new pamphlet, advertisement to buy a new book review, cassette, video, RTL newspaper, a message/letter from the national office, newsletter every day without exception a tie to the work, a movie, video, even People magazine in the Safeway. I was always aware that abortions were proceeding relentlessly somewhere in this world. I never let myself forget. I was connected like people with Ipods, I guess, or an internet junky, but long before widespread internet access. I also had visuals, listening to tapes, etc, for example, a testimony of Dr. Hern to abortionists on how he performed a D&C abortion from a catholic newspaper.

Another way I was able to endure the struggle with my feelings of incompetence was the daily contact with staff. I didn't work every day but I called in to talk to the volunteer on duty. I visited the office often after Mass in the morning besides my shifts. I always worked from home but as the years went by I saw that much more was needed in the face of growing numbers of Birthright Centers. I was not Director all 35 years. There were a series of Directors from 1975-1982: Jackie Hanigan, Lucy Berg, Sandy Schmidt, Joyce Locke, and Suzy Stores. We always talked but during those years I felt more detached from the daily workings. I did my shift but I didn't appreciate how profoundly our work with the women was affecting the outcomes of their pregnancy. I was busy with my young and growing family and school and sports activities overshadowed a lot of the vision the intensity I feel now just was a lot less then.

In 1982 things changed dramatically when the series of Directors was exhausted. I realized that someone had to take charge in a more consistent way. Abortion numbers were at their all time peak. Our little 400 square foot office was bustling with clients but the encounter on one afternoon shift made me realize a truly painful reality and I started to change. The woman in front of me was lovely, well dressed and put together but was so desperate to keep her man. She discovered through hiding in his apartment and listening to a conversation on his phone with another woman that she would be totally alone in this pregnancy. What she heard from her hiding place shocked her. He was planning to dump her!

Recounting the knowledge was a truly awful moment for both of us in different ways. She, so dependent upon him to go to such lengths to find out the truth and I, watching her tear stained face and witnessing a human being disintegrating, crumbling before me because of such tremendous distress! I could not forget this woman and while I could not help her as I would have liked (she went ahead with the abortion), I thought about her and could not forget her desperation. This moved me to try harder to be a better, more attentive worker in this movement. Paradoxically, the feelings of incompetence seemed to fade. I forgot about my preoccupation with my efforts and effects. It was not a conscious decision, however. Looking back, I just forgot about myself and just started to focus everything in me on this one particular woman in front of me during our encounter.

During this renewed process of years of training at meetings, reading lectures; on my own, together with less self-criticism, I found St. Therese, The Little Flower who said, "If you are willing to bear serenely the trial of being displeasing to yourself, then you will be for Jesus a pleasant place of shelter" (Schmidt, 2006). One by one, my children left home for college. I had a lot more time to focus on the work. I started a Regional newsletter. I called center directors on the phone. I wrote more letters to other consultants asking how they worked out problems like advertising and counseling. I planned our staff meetings with more care, and found worthwhile speakers in our community such as Jack Harrington.

Another great help to me personally was to develop other interests, now that my children were leaving the nest. My mother had always encouraged me to continue my education. When she died I took up the challenge once again and enrolled in the University of Oregon in Italian. I had lived in Italy for a time and love all things Italian. My sorrow was that I couldn't speak the language so I took a first course in Romance Language Dept for one trimester each year. Then, the desire just grew to learn more so I ended up with three trimesters a year for many years. It continues. The joy of hearing, speaking and learning the politics, arts, etc. of Italy has sustained me and been a wonderful counterpoint to the harsh reality of abortions on demand. It has widened my vision of the world and through my friendship with an Italian counterpart in Viareggio I have been comforted that there are people, ordinary housewives, all over the world who want to fight abortion and help pregnant women.

Another step in my determination to keep working is the fact that I became a grandmother in 1984. I honestly don't consider myself a good mother. I was too nervous and distracted by the duties and responsibilities but being a grandmother is a good fit for me. I am much more relaxed, less demanding, and more accepting. I want to help these dear children.

During 1994 there were two big losses for pro-life, one very close to us. Joe McCullough, the lawyer for NLC Board, died suddenly. He was a big support to all of us on the USA Board, sort of a fatherly strong presence. Another, Dr. Jerome LeJeune was a world famous fetalogist, whom I had met in Russia. His thoughtful and thought-provoking defense for the preservation of seven human embryos at his testimony given at a divorce trial showed that the extraordinary uniqueness of each human baby with a distinct DNA like the code of packages at the supermarket was to be recognized and respected. Out of the millions of possibilities for human beings only one.

There are always new challenges. Currently our next-door neighbors at the office will not allow us to use our sandwich board on our shared sidewalk. Another nearby neighbor, Planned Parenthood, reminds us daily that there is still work to be done. Most important of all, abortions to 23 weeks are still done right here in Eugene, two days each week.

After decades of abortion on demand we now have the concern not only of the lost children, but also for the mothers who have experienced abortion. These women must be met with hope and not condemnation. They have often been lied to and have suffered great psychological and spiritual trauma due to their experience with abortion.

In the 1990s the Holy Father John Paul II wrote these words in the encyclical *Evangelum Vitae*:

> I would now like to say a special word to women
> who have had an abortion. The Church is aware of
> the many factors which may have influenced your

decision, and she does not doubt that in many cases it was a painful and even shattering decision. The wound in your heart may not yet have healed. Certainly what happened was and remains terribly wrong. But do not give in to discouragement and do not lose hope. Try rather to understand what happened and face it honestly. If you have not already done so, give yourselves over with humility and trust to repentance. The Father of mercies is ready to give you His peace in the Sacrament of Reconciliation. You will come to understand that nothing is definitively lost and you will also be able to ask forgiveness from your child, who is now living in the Lord. With the friendly and expert help and advice of other people, and as a result of your own painful experience, you can be among the most eloquent defenders of everyone's right to life. Through your commitment to life, whether by accepting the birth of other children or by welcoming and caring for those most in need of someone to be close to them, you will become promoters of a new way of looking at human life (John Paul II, 1995).

Just as John Paul II calls the women who have experienced abortion to be sources of hope, I too strive to be a promoter of a new way of looking at human life. This is ultimately the goal that brings me strength and hope. Looking back through the years I am amazed at the endurance God has granted me in the face of this great evil, abortion. Even today there are clear reasons to continue working and hoping as volunteers and organizations across the country remain steadfast in the cause of life.

CHAPTER 5.

New Workers in the Field: Evangelicals and Others

Before the mid 1980s the primary religious support for the pro-life movement came from the Catholic Church. Although she had been roundly criticized and ridiculed for her stance supporting life, there was little alliance or support from other groups for the decade 1973-1983. However, the Evangelical community was largely awakened and stirred into action by the 1979 film followed by the book in 1983 titled, *Whatever Happened to the Human Race*, by Francis Schaefer and Dr. C. Everett Koop (Koop & Schaefer, 1983). These men urged their fellow evangelicals to get into the fight against abortion. Following this new awareness the Evangelical community began to fervently embrace the pregnancy care movement.

Evangelical minister, Curtis Young, formed a group called the Christian Action Council, CAC. By the mid 1980s, as the stalwart leader of the CAC, Curt Young, a practical man, and ordained minister, added the purpose of spreading the gospel message to the pregnant women who came for help. He was very keen, indeed, to transform the Birthright model into an arm of the Christian Church. Thus the pregnancy service movement could bring these needy families to a saving knowledge of Jesus Christ. The distinction from the Birthright system is that, though many Birthright centers are supported by local Christian leaders and many workers are Christian, no evangelization is allowed and no religious affiliation is claimed for the centers as a whole.

The CAC and its many affiliates are now known under the umbrella name of CareNet and share in the struggle to support pregnant women. Today these groups are composed mostly of dedicated evangelicals. They offer help as Birthright centers do: tests, clothing, counseling and generally follow a similar pro-life program. I believe there will always be a need for compassionate friends who can be available to the pregnant woman who faces so many difficulties in carrying her baby to term.

Following the split in the Birthright organization in 1993, our center became an affiliate of the National Life Center run by Denise Cocciolone under the new name of 1st Way. Soon after, many different names were used by former Birthright centers in the U.S. including Aurora, Birth Choice, and Birthline. No longer having the unity of the Birthright Charter, meant that many centers now were no longer united in purpose as well. In the 1970s there were only 2 models, Birthright and AAI. Now there are hundreds even thousands of centers with different names. Some of these reflect the expansion of the mission, for example, including adoptions and abstinence. Some have added more medical assistance such as ultrasounds and STD testing. There are at least four or five national hotlines that can now be accessed by women in need.

Sharing the Birthright name supported branding and name recognition across the country. Losing that has been a challenge. There are not very many 1st Way centers and so name recognition is poor. The great variety of names reflects the variety in missions as well. In some ways this jeopardizes the original vision of a pregnancy center. One does not know now when one calls if the center will only emphasize alternatives to abortion or will promote additional agendas. Our 1st Way has maintained the original vision of Louise Summerhill's Charter, though not necessarily that of the Birthright program since her passing. For example, ultrasound offers a window to the womb that helps women see their options other than abortion, yet the use of this technology is not permitted at Birthright centers.

About 15 years ago, the Lane Pregnancy Support Services Director, Jeanie Langley, Feminists for Life Chair in Eugene, Kathy Freeman and I attempted to meet on a semi-regular basis. With only a few encounters under our belts the meetings simply dried up. Why, I don't know. We had some minor disagreements, such as a TV commercial from Vitae Co. that was due to be screened locally. I thought they were subtle and sophisticated, but Jeanie felt they would not be beneficial. Such disagreement was not the norm, however, and I very much missed our little gatherings where there was a sense of understanding and compassion towards each other. Kathy Freeman, member of Feminists for Life, dropped our meetings. Not that she didn't support the cause, but because of growing family commitments, including a new baby and back to work issues. The LPSS staff has continued to work with local pro-life groups on the annual Parade for Life on the birthday of Roe, Jan 22.

I am willing to admit that sometimes there has occasionally been a feeling of competition among the various CPCs as well as the LPSS. This is only evidence of the human side of those who do this work, including me. However, I do not sit and pine for the old days with the well organized structure of the Birthright system. Rather I have pursued connections to other CPCs regardless of affiliation. After all, our mission is a shared one. Though not everyone is equally open to such connections, I have met with almost all the other CareNet centers around the State of Oregon, with mostly positive response and we have helped each other. For example, the center in Lebanon was very helpful in solving some of 1st Way's ultrasound problems. I have also traveled to various CareNet centers for regional meetings.

Another joint venture that has lasted and been more fruitful has been the initiation on the part of Corvallis Pregnancy Center of a web site, PossiblyPregnant.org. From that initial step in to the world of the web there were at least 2 get-togethers I attended with board members. The webmaster, Jeff Jimerson, remains very open to suggestions from the local members. My center added its own Hispanic-looking woman and our own stories of pregnant women clients and how they were helped by 1st Way. The web site now has 11 centers and has an active participation with many "hits." Clients have come or called our office because of the site. Now there is even some money to help with advertising like billboards, etc. This pleases me because it means I am not alone.

The Birthright in Salem, headed by my dear friend, Terry Brand, also attests to the friendly cooperation among the five crisis pregnancy centers in Salem. Terry is an outstanding administrator. She also has a true commitment to the unborn and a womanly instinct for nurturing pregnant women. Staying in touch with Terry and these nearby centers further supports our own 1st Way center in Eugene, because again, we are not alone.

Happily, I have been able to share my own knowledge and experience in ultrasound with the St. Germaine center in Salem. In 2004 we pooled our resources and invited Shari Richard, a professional ultrasound teacher to come for an in-service for our techs to learn about the latest sonogram techniques. All ultrasounds are overseen by our medical director, yet outside training by a sonogram specialist was still a great help for our technicians. This extra professional education has benefited both centers in Eugene and Salem. The St. Germaine center is right next door to the largest Planned Parenthood campus in Oregon, maybe in the whole USA.

In addition, during the ultrasound classes, we were able to share our overflow of maternity clothes at one point as well. This reminded me of the early days where all Birthright centers would share not only their clients problems but also the material wealth of trendy maternity clothing. Loads and loads were exchanged to bolster the closets of our respective centers.

This type of benefit only came by working together. For example, whenever a regional Birthright meeting was scheduled, husbands, sons, and friends were recruited to load up the cars with maternity clothing to exchange during these gatherings. These meetings were gatherings of the troops to reinforce and replenish our spirits, to get to know one another better and to learn about the needs and benefits of various state policies of our union. Such meetings were in part made possible by the charter system which gave us common goals and a system of leadership across the country. Even so, I have previously discussed the difficulties of getting all the Birthright directors to follow similar protocols in pursuit of our common goals. Pro-lifers are indeed independent personalities, so attempts to work together without a common charter and a regional network of leadership can be an even greater challenge.

Nonetheless, it is my goal to continue to foster relationships between 1st Way and all other CPCs regardless of religious background. We must remain as united as possible in our goals and support one another; divided we will fall.

Chapter 6.

Hope for the Future

When I and so many others across the country began to combat the specter of abortion by supporting the needs of pregnant women, we were introduced to a side of the heart of Christ, the sorrowful side which grieves for the destruction of His creation. We could not ignore the visible evidence of God's creative Hand in the unborn babies, babies all around us everyday so banal, a baby, yet so precious, so crucial to all human existence.

Our faith in God's intentional purpose in the workings of the wonderful human body deepened. Pregnancy and birth are truly mysteries, miracles of intricacy and complexity; the meaning usually escapes our conscious awareness but we can understand hope. Hope is the source of blessing and joy. A new child is the fulfillment of hope; the real come into our history.

If someone were to try to characterize the CPC workers as people who are trying to bring the Kingdom of God into history, he would be met with a quizzical look. Such lofty terms escape our daily perception because our work is patchy, three hours once a week, giving tests, folding clothes, and answering telephones. We are from the middle class, women with husbands and children, shoppers at Safeway, members of PTAs, cooks and housekeepers for our families. We do have a vision; it is the joyful relationship of mother and child. The vision we have in the midst of the desperate plight of the distressed pregnant woman is sometimes obscured and shattered by the utter foolish dependency on boyfriends or non-appreciation of the contents of the pregnant uterus. But God's intentional purpose is always toward the wonder of the human body. It is truly a mystery; the intricacy and complexity and the meaning escapes our conscious comprehension. Yet we can understand hope as a source of blessing and reality come into our very history. Even critics have grasped the scope of our work:

In their quiet way the crisis pregnancy centers and post-abortion recovery groups represent a dimension of the anti-abortion movement that is passionate and far reaching, consisting not of protesters or political activists but of Christian therapy groups, crisis pregnancy centers, adoption agencies and support programs for single mothers and their children (Leland, 2006).

Our passion is far reaching, yet it only needs to reach as far as the individual woman. We eschew political intrigues for the real action instead. We meet mothers where they are, where they need.

Lately we are finding that our service movement is turning more professional. Many centers now pay an executive director full time along with an ultrasound technician, nurses and an administrative assistant. Even some 1st Way centers have followed this trend, though not yet here in Eugene. This increases the need for additional fundraising, which can be a significant strain. Perhaps the paid staff will improve the services offered by CPCs, but perhaps not. I can only suggest that the memory of the original Birthright center must somehow be preserved along with the new technology. In her book, *Building Resiliency*, Mary Lyn Pulley (2002) suggests that "long term volunteers are one of the ways that organizations preserve a corporate memory; without these old timers and their memories, how can we store the knowledge of our original vision, one that accumulates values and uses the knowledge." The memory of the CPC organization's history produces a specific culture of personal and truthful friendship, both among workers and with the women who come to us.

Whether that can be maintained by paid professionals, I don't know. But I believe the original vision is worth saving. That memory is in us, the long term volunteers. As we proceed further in the Twenty-first

Century I have committed myself to writing this book in order to honor the singular group of people who gave birth to this movement and tended to its needs in the early years. We sweated it out, day after day and year after year, bequeathing the stories of struggle and their memories to all those who have and will continue to join in along the way.

There is plenty more for new hearts and hands to contribute. Some CPCs, such as Expectant Mothers Care, a CPC operating in the Bronx, have begun to meet the needs of more women through the use of a converted RV for mobile pregnancy tests and ultrasounds. With the advent of the Internet, pregnant women can just click on abortion and find names, addresses of abortion providers in their vicinity. Without even going to an office, an abortion appointment can be made on line. Furthermore, RU 486 and other emergency contraception options make "do it yourself" abortions an ever present reality. Statistics tell us that abortion rates are down but they cannot measure how much may be due to the use of chemicals to cause abortion like Plan B and RU 486. How to meet these challenges is God's work for younger hands.

It is crucial to remember that even in the climate of private options, most women desire to talk about their problems with one whom they trust. That is why CPCs were created and that is why we are here and why we will still be here in the future. I know that God is with us and that there is always hope.

Bibliography

Banducci, Marian. (2003). *Twenty Years on the Front Lines*. Published by Voice for the Unborn.

Carlo Cassini. (1974). *Leaves for Life*. Eurostampa Periodici Italiani.

Crutcher, Mark. (1996). *Lime 5: Exploited by Choice*. Denton, TX: Life Dynamics, Inc.

Drogin, Elasah. (1979). *Margaret Sanger: Father of Modern Society*. New Hope, KY: CUL Publishers.

Ellis, Haveloch. (1911). *The Problem of Race Regeneration*. New York: Moffat, Yard & Co.

Ensor, J. (2003). *Answering the Call: Saving Innocent Lives, One Woman at a Time*. Carol Stream, IL: Tyndale House Publishers.

Erlich, P. (1968). *The Population Bomb*. Sierra Club/Ballantine.

Fairchild, Henry Pratt. (1977). *The Melting Pot Mistake*. New York: Arno Press,

Faludi, Susan. (1991). *Backlash: The Undeclared War Against American Women*. New York: Doubleday.

Fitzgerald, Maureen. (2006). *Habits of Compassion: Irish Catholic Nuns and the Origins of the Welfare System, 1830-1920*. Chicago: University of Illinois Press.

Garton, Jean Staker. (1979). *Who Broke the Baby?* Bethany Fellowship, Minneapolis, MN.

Gaskin, Ina May. (1975, 1977, 1980, 1990, 2002). *Spiritual Midwifery*. Summertown, TN: Book Publishing Co.

Hartshom, Margaret. (2009, Jan. 17). *Back to the Drawing Board*. St. Augustine's Press, World; Abortion Past.

Hendershott, Anne. (2006). *The Politics of Abortion*. New York: Encounter Books.

John Paul II. (1995). *Evangelium Vitae: On the value and inviolability of human life*. Encyclical Letter. Washington, D. C.: United States Catholic Conference.

Koop, C. Everett, & Schaefer, F. (1983). *Whatever Happened to the Human Race*, by Crossway Books, 1983. Movie released by Gospel Communications, January, 1979.

Leland, John. (2006, June 16). Compassionate Alternatives. *New York Times*.

Mannion, Michael T. (1996). *Abortion and Healing: A Cry to Be Whole*. Franklin, WI: Sheed & Ward.

Mathews-Greens, Frederica. (1994). *Real Choices*. Multnomah Books.

Nathanson, Bernard. (1981). *Aborting America*. Edinburgh: Pinnacle Books.

O'Conner, F. (2008, May). *Voices*, XXIII(2).

Powell, John, SJ. (1981). *The Silent Holocaust*. Allen, TX: Argus Communications.

Pulley, Mary Lynn. ((2002). *Building Resiliency: How to Thrive in Times of Change*. Greensboro, NC: Center For Creative Leadership.

Riley, Patrick J. A book review in "Emmanuel" of *Habits of Compassion*. Minn Ursuline College, Peppertree.

Schmidt, Joseph. (2006). *Everything in Grace*. Ijamsville, MD: The Word Among Us Press.

Seuss, T. (1954). *Horton Hears a Who*. New York: Random House.

Simon, David, & Burns, Edward. (1997). *The Corner: A Year in the Life of Inner City Neighborhoods*. Broadway Books.

Summerhill, Louise. (1968). *The story of Birthright*. Kenosha, WS: Prow Books.

Thompson, L. (1994). *Mastering the Challenges of Change*. New York: Amacom.

Verney, Thomas. (1981). *The Secret Life of the Unborn Child*. New York: Dell Books.

Wilke, John. (1971). *Handbook on Abortion*. Cincinnati: Hayes Publishing Co.

www.ingramcontent.com/pod-product-compliance
Lightning Source LLC
Chambersburg PA
CBHW020255290526
45784CB00003B/1265